D0017029

LANDMARK

LANDMARK

*The Inside Story of
America's New Health-Care Law
and What It Means for Us All*

THE STAFF OF

The Washington Post

PublicAffairs
New York

Copyright © 2010 by The Washington Post.

Published in the United States by PublicAffairs™, a member of the Perseus Books Group. All rights reserved.

Printed in the United States of America.

No part of this book may be reproduced in any manner whatsoever without written permission except in the case of brief quotations embodied in critical articles and reviews. For information, address PublicAffairs, 250 West 57th Street, Suite 1321, New York, NY 10107.

PublicAffairs books are available at special discounts for bulk purchases in the U.S. by corporations, institutions, and other organizations. For more information, please contact the Special Markets Department at the Perseus Books Group, 2300 Chestnut Street, Suite 200, Philadelphia, PA 19103, call (800) 810-4145, ext. 5000, or e-mail special.markets@perseusbooks.com.

Text set in Adobe Caslon

Cataloging-in-Publication Data is available from the Library of Congress
ISBN: 978-1-58648-934-2

First Edition

10 9 8 7 6 5 4 3 2 1

CONTENTS

v

FOREWORD

For more than a century, Americans have debated whether and how to extend health care across society. While politicians argued about what was desirable and what was possible, advances in medicine eradicated diseases, extended life spans and transformed our quality of life.

But there was a cost, and it was vast. Nearly one in every six dollars spent in the world's most powerful economy went to health care. Yet nearly one in every six people went without coverage that would ensure their access to medical care. The imperative for change loomed ever larger.

In March 2010, Congress acted. The Patient Protection and Affordable Care Act, narrowly passed after a raucous, bitterly partisan debate, will bring about the broadest transformation of the health-care system in this country since Medicare and Medicaid were created nearly half a century ago. Love it or hate it—and the nation is as riven as Congress was—the new law will have an immense impact.

It requires nearly every American to carry health insurance. It compels insurers to cover new clients, even those who are already ill. It alters the way millions of people will shop for insurance. It enlarges some government programs and cuts back on others. For the wealthy, some taxes will rise. For the poor, new subsidies will be available. The government's role in the largest sector of our economy will grow.

It took lawmakers 2,073 pages, before adjustments in a separate follow-up bill, to draft the new architecture of health care in the United States. This book is designed to make sense of it, to put the legalisms into plain English and to explain how they affect us all— you, your family, your doctors, hospitals, insurance companies and many other component parts of this sprawling industry. It also contains an extraordinary behind-the-scenes account of the political calculations and compromises that made the law possible.

The Washington Post has committed dozens of reporters, graphic artists, editors and other news staffers to coverage of the health-care debate over the past year. Two writers in particular deserve mention. Ceci Connolly reported the inside narrative over many months, informed by interviews with key participants. Alec MacGillis closely followed the development of the legislation and used his expertise to frame this guidebook.

We and our partners at PublicAffairs are pleased to offer you this fascinating tale and invaluable primer to understanding a landmark change in American policy. Whether you welcome or rue the new law, this book is essential reading.

MARCUS BRAUCHLI
Executive Editor
The Washington Post

INTRODUCTION

By Dan Balz

On March 23, 2010, President Barack Obama, using 22 pens, signed the Patient Protection and Affordable Care Act. The import of the ceremony in the East Room of the White House was lost on neither those who supported the measure nor those who had vigorously opposed it. Congressional approval of health-care reform marked the most significant advance in health-care policy since passage of Medicare and Medicaid in 1965. In terms of social welfare legislation, it also ranked alongside the enactment of Social Security in 1935. With his signature, Obama had put his presidency in the history books.

"We are a nation that faces its challenges and accepts its responsibilities," he told the audience. "We are a nation that does what is hard. What is necessary. What is right. Here, in this country, we shape our own destiny. That is what we do. That is who we are. That is what makes us the United States of America. And we have now just enshrined . . . the core principle that everybody should have some basic security when it comes to their health care. And it is an extraordinary achievement."

For all the sense of excitement that accompanied the signing ceremony, there was a parallel reality. The health-care bill divided Americans like few other issues in recent memory. Passage came after one of the longest, most rancorous and most partisan debates the capital has seen in years. In pressing for broad reform, the president not only made history, he also put the Democratic Party at risk.

The debate raged for a year. It gave rise to a grass-roots movement of activists who became known as "tea partiers" and conjured up fears of encroaching big government, sparked angry protests at town hall meetings and tested the capacity of a new president and Democratic majorities in Congress to deliver on their loftiest promises. At times, the legislation appeared stalled. At other times, it was on life support, particularly in the days after a little-known Republican named Scott Brown captured the Massachusetts Senate seat held for more than 40 years by the late Edward M. Kennedy, a Democrat whose name was associated so strongly with the cause of providing health-care coverage to all Americans. In the end, the legislation passed without a single Republican vote—a far different outcome than for Medicare or Social Security, which ultimately enjoyed bipartisan majorities.

This book chronicles how ideas that had been in the public realm for a century finally became the law of the land, and what it will mean for every person in the country. Americans who wonder how Obama succeeded where so many other presidents failed will find the inside story of the legislative struggle, with all its drama, a compelling narrative of Washington in action. Those who want to know what the fine print in the 2,000-page document (plus the reconciliation bill that cleaned up some of the worst backroom deals) really says can find the answers in these pages. Those who want to read the official summary themselves will also find that in this book.

The account here is the latest chapter in a much longer and richer story. Providing health insurance for all citizens was a goal enunciated early in the 20th century by Theodore Roosevelt. For the past eight decades, many presidents sought to fulfill that vision. Most of them were Democrats, but a few were Republicans. With each effort, a fierce debate erupted, a clash that reflects some of the most deep-seated philosophical questions that have divided the republic since its founding: What is the proper role of government? What is the relationship between government and individuals? What kind of social safety net should government provide to its citizens? Which services are best left to free markets and which warrant federal intervention? Which responsibilities should be given to the federal government and which to the states? And, always, what can the country afford?

Those debates, repeated time and again, were both high-minded and given to extremes. With each effort to expand the system came charges of socialism, socialized medicine and at times talk of Soviet-style health care or the Europeanization of America. Obama faced those accusations as well as others, including the spurious claim that his legislation would establish death panels that would have the power to decide whether Grandma and Grandpa lived or died.

As has often been said, health care is both the most personal and the most complex public policy issue, and the passions it arouses are understandable. To succeed, proponents of reform have had to fight off powerful special interests from the industry, from the American Medical Association to the hospital lobby to the insurance and drug companies. No wonder so many presidents tried without success; no wonder that, even with passage this time, the debate continues to boil across the country.

Congress has played a central role in every great battle over health-care reform, but it is presidents who matter most. In their 2009 book, *The Heart of Power: Health and Politics in the Oval Office*, David Blumenthal, a Harvard professor (who is an official in the Department of Health and Human Services), and James A. Morone of Brown University wrote: "Major health care reform is virtually impossible: difficult to understand, swarming with interests, powered by money and resonating with popular anxiety. The first key to success is a president who cares about it deeply. Only a president with real commitment will invest in such a dangerous and risky venture. It costs time, energy and political capital. This is no arena for half-hearted efforts."

Although Theodore Roosevelt is given credit for starting the country on a course toward national health insurance, his contribution was actually modest and fleeting. His embrace of the idea came not while he was in the White House as the Republican Party's standard-bearer but later, during his unsuccessful bid for the presidency in 1912 as the Progressive Party's nominee. The party platform included one sentence calling for "the protection of home life against the hazards of sickness, irregular employment and old age through the adoption of a system of social insurance adapted to American use." Roosevelt lost that election to Woodrow Wilson.

For two decades, the idea languished, until Franklin D. Roosevelt was elected in 1932 in the depths of the Great Depression. Roosevelt was a great social crusader, the New Deal architect who redefined the relationship between government and the economy and was elected four times. While he embraced the concept of providing health insurance for all Americans, he was never willing to put the rest of his agenda at risk for the cause. He considered it in 1935, as part of a grand economic security initiative, a bill that would include Social Security and unemployment insurance. But he pulled healthcare reform out before sending the measure to Congress, fearing it might sink the entire package. He considered it twice more during his presidency. In one case, he blinked again, as he had done in 1935. The last effort ended with Roosevelt's death in 1945.

Harry S. Truman picked up the mantle from Roosevelt. He was, if anything, more committed to the cause of national health insurance than Roosevelt, pledging only four months after FDR's death to send Congress a plan. But Truman never pushed hard for health care. Republican victories in the 1946 elections then doomed chances of congressional action. Truman kept proposing, but the pattern repeated itself. Even after he unexpectedly won election in 1948, he supported comprehensive health-care reform but did not make it a top priority. As Democrats backed away, they shifted focus to a more modest goal: health care for the elderly, or what later would be known as Medicare.

There was no significant progress on comprehensive health-care legislation under Republican Dwight D. Eisenhower. He resisted efforts to broaden the government's role, preferring to find ways to strengthen private insurance. He initially opposed Medicare legislation in Congress, then toward the end of his presidency came around. It was too late.

Still, two important changes occurred during his administration. One was the creation of the Federal Employees Health Benefits Program, which in recent years became the model that all politicians cited as the kind of insurance options all Americans should have. The other was a change of enormous significance: the expansion and institutionalization of the tax break for employer-sponsored health insurance—a provision that costs the government more than $150 billion annually and that was fiercely fought over in the latest health-care battle as a new source of revenue to pay for expanded coverage.

Democrat John F. Kennedy championed Medicare during his shortened presidency. He came close to winning in 1962, only to see the legislation die after one senator switched sides in a back-room deal similar to the infamous "Cornhusker Kickback" that Sen. Ben Nelson, a Nebraska Democrat, won in return for his vote for health-care legislation in December 2009. But in Kennedy's time it was used to defeat the bill, not salvage it.

Lyndon B. Johnson finally succeeded, although it took two tries. The Democrat nearly got a Medicare bill out of Congress in 1964, only to see it wither late in the term. Then, backed by huge Democratic majorities that grew out of his 1964 landslide and with a command of the legislative process virtually unrivaled in the modern presidency, he pushed again. By the summer of 1965, he had his victory: legislation that created both Medicare and Medicaid. Johnson signed the bill in Truman's home town of Independence, Missouri. "You have made me a very happy man," Truman told Johnson. "I'm glad to have lived this long." Johnson gave Truman the first pen used to sign the bill.

Richard M. Nixon is best remembered for the Watergate scandal and his overture to China. But the Republican made a major and lasting contribution to the health-care debate that carried forward to Obama's presidency. With Ted Kennedy pushing from the left for national insurance, Nixon felt pressure to respond with his own plan. In his 1974 State of the Union address, he proposed comprehensive health-care reform. Drawing a distinction with Kennedy's vision, which Nixon said would put the system under the "heavy hand of government," he called for building on the existing framework of employer-based insurance and proposed legislation that included a mandate on employers to offer coverage. Nixon's architecture formed the basis for what Obama would pursue three decades later. As impeachment closed in on Nixon, his administration continued to negotiate with Kennedy in hopes of reaching a compromise. Nixon's resignation in August 1974 brought those negotiations to a halt.

Kennedy, however, did not abandon the cause, and his determination to press for national health insurance split the Democratic Party during Jimmy Carter's presidency. Carter was not wedded to national coverage and he clashed with Kennedy over what should be done. That led to the senator's unsuccessful challenge to Carter in the 1980 Democratic primaries. Carter, weakened by the divisions within his party, but even more by the Iranian hostage crisis, was defeated by Republican Ronald Reagan in the general election.

Reagan's presidency produced a major expansion of Medicare—catastrophic coverage for senior citizens that he proposed—and a prescription drug benefit added by the Democrats. But a revolt among many of those older Americans over new taxes that would pay for the change forced Congress to repeal the law early in the presidency of Republican George H.W. Bush.

It was left to the next Democratic president, Bill Clinton, to take up the battle once again for comprehensive insurance. Health-care reform was a central part of Clinton's campaign in 1992, but he was slow to move the legislation to Congress. When he did, he delivered a massive and complicated bill written virtually in secret under the direction of his wife, Hillary Rodham Clinton, and health adviser Ira Magaziner. The bill provoked widespread opposition, particularly from the health-care industry, which sponsored the effective "Harry and Louise" ads that helped stymie Congress. The effort ended disastrously for the Democrats: The measure never came to a vote on the floor of either chamber, and Republicans won control of the House and Senate in the 1994 midterm elections.

Clinton's debacle set back the cause for more than a decade but did not stop major changes in health policy. Republican George W. Bush signed the biggest expansion of Medicare since its enactment: a prescription drug benefit. But it was not until the 2008 presidential election that major Democratic candidates once again robustly embraced the concept of universal health-care reform, with Obama, Hillary Clinton and John Edwards all producing plans for comprehensive coverage.

Of the three, Obama's was the most conservative, eschewing any requirement that all Americans buy insurance. His rivals questioned his commitment to universal coverage. When Kennedy endorsed Obama in January 2008, he asked in return that Obama pledge to make health-care reform his top domestic priority and commit himself to the goal of universal coverage.

Obama readily agreed, and 26 months later—14 months after his inauguration—he fulfilled that promise. He proved highly flexible in his efforts to win congressional approval, even changing his mind about the need for an individual mandate, which he had vigorously opposed as a candidate. He and his team, drawing on mistakes from Clinton's presidency, allowed Congress considerable leeway to write the legislation (too much, said many critics). They also worked assiduously to keep the health-care industry at the table throughout the debate in an effort to prevent the kind of opposition that had killed the Clinton plan. "Our presence here today," he said in the East Room when he signed the legislation, "is remarkable and improbable."

The debate did not end with Obama's signature. The latest battle will continue to play out in the elections of 2010 and 2012. It will resurface as the new law is implemented in stages and, likely, as future Congresses consider changes. The legislation represents a major milestone in the ongoing discussion about health care in the United States but, as history tells us, not the last word.

PART I

HOW WE GOT HERE

By Ceci Connolly

CHAPTER 1

The Call of History: "We're Gonna Get This Done"

Barack Obama shifted uncomfortably from one foot to the other.

Two months after announcing his run for the presidency, the junior senator from Illinois was standing on a stage in Las Vegas on the morning of March 24, 2007, facing hundreds of Democratic activists.

He had flown halfway across the country late the night before to be there. The event was a candidate forum on health care, and several of his opponents had dazzled the crowd.

Hillary Rodham Clinton, who had struggled hard for a health-care bill in 1993 during her husband's presidency, proved she knew more about the complicated subject than anyone in the hall.

John Edwards, appearing with his wife days after announcing that her cancer had returned, moved them with his fervor.

But when Obama's turn came, it quickly became apparent that this man who would be president had little to say.

"Everybody on this stage is going to have a plan to move this health-care debate forward," he offered. "I will be putting out a plan over the next couple of months."

He spoke tentatively and in vague generalities, and when one person in the audience said she couldn't find much on the Internet about his views on health-care policy, he struck a defensive note.

11

"Keep in mind that our campaign now is, I think, a little over eight weeks old," he replied. Perhaps she hadn't looked in the right place, he suggested. "I'm not sure whether you're going to the campaign Web site or my Senate Web site," he said.

But the young woman said she had checked both. The fact was, there just wasn't much there, and as he finished speaking, two of the most prominent leaders in modern Democratic Party politics, seated beside each other in the front row, wondered whether Obama was ready to be a first-tier candidate.

"That was a little flat," thought Andy Stern, president of the Service Employees International Union, surprised that the man known for stirring oratory was so lackluster.

"I was expecting the crowd to be with him," John Podesta, president of the Center for American Progress and Bill Clinton's former chief of staff, remarked to Stern.

Eventually, both men would become ardent backers of Obama. So, too, would Sen. Edward M. Kennedy (D-Mass.), the liberal giant who had made universal health care his lifelong mission. Obama would find his voice on the issue, ascend to the presidency, and make health-care reform a central goal of his administration.

But on that day in March 2007, no one—not even Obama— saw history in the making.

While many of the other candidates stayed after the event to work the crowd, Obama drove straight to the airport. On the telephone with his campaign manager, he gave a clear-eyed self-critique.

"I just whiffed up there," he told David Plouffe.

That was his diagnosis. Next came his cure:

"We need a plan," he continued. "And obviously we're gonna have a plan."

*   *   *

Three years after his dismal performance in Las Vegas, Obama accomplished what no president for decades had been able to achieve: enactment of landmark legislation that guarantees health care to nearly every American.

Shortly before midnight on March 21, 2010, Congress approved the sprawling bill and Obama told the nation: "Tonight, we answered the call of history."

How did he go from fumbling in Las Vegas to making history in the White House? What prompted a new president to tackle an issue for which he was not particularly known? And why, months later, was he willing to stake his presidency on such a complex and controversial piece of legislation?

To some extent, he didn't have much choice. "Health care for all" has been the mantra of liberal constituencies for nearly a century, and any Democratic politician with national aspirations must pay homage to the cause. He also felt bound by his promises, first to Kennedy, and then to voters, to make the issue a top priority.

Still, Obama could have set more modest goals, as some urged. Several administration economists argued that it was risky in a recession to pursue a costly government expansion. Vice President Biden and White House Chief of Staff Rahm Emanuel, both of whom had served in Congress, feared that lawmakers couldn't process Obama's already ambitious agenda, which included an economic stimulus package, education reform, and bailouts for banks and automakers.

But the new president became convinced that rising medical costs were crippling average families, cutting into corporate profits and consuming more and more of the federal budget. If he did not slow the exorbitant increases, little money would be left for anything else.

Thus Obama, viewing himself as a transformational figure, instructed his team to map out an aggressive plan for refashioning one-sixth of the nation's economy.

Those were his reasons for trying. The story of how he accomplished it is one of the great Washington tales, a story that in the end is not so much about health care as it is about the way the nation's capital works.

In the 14 months from his inauguration to the March 23, 2010, bill-signing ceremony in the East Room of the White House, Obama's quest vacillated from the mundane to the epic. It was an odyssey marked by clashing egos and bitter betrayals, of unexpected detours and roadblocks. More than once, it nearly died.

Many of the protagonists were reprising roles they'd played 15 years earlier, when Bill Clinton had tried to overhaul the health-care system and failed. Before Clinton's failure had been Carter's. Before Carter's had been Nixon's. So it had gone, back in time, for decades.

But with his high popularity ratings, his Democratic Party in control of Congress and a failing economy that sparked unease among the middle class about rising medical costs, Obama believed he could achieve the improbable. "The stars are aligned," he liked to say.

At times, the president seemed so far removed from the action that loyalists accused him of abandoning a fundamental campaign pledge. At other moments, he became not only the lead salesman, but the chief dealmaker as well.

"I am not the first president to take up this cause, but I am determined to be the last," he said in a joint address to Congress in September 2009.

In the Internet era, much of the saga played out in real time, in public view. Legislative machinations and partisan spin were chronicled daily by the mainstream media and chewed over minute by minute in the blogosphere. In all, about $1 billion was spent on lobbying and advertising. Much more happened behind closed doors, where strategy was hatched, deals struck, promises made and threats hurled.

The full impact of the law—a major reworking of the nation's $2.4 trillion-a-year health-care system—will not be known for years, if not decades. By 2014, every American will be required to carry health insurance, though tens of millions will receive it for free or at a discount. Senior citizens will pay less for medication, wealthy people will face higher taxes, insurers will be subject to stricter regulations, and doctors and hospitals will be under financial pressure to improve the quality of care. How will it all work out?

The political implications are even harder to project. Immediately after the legislation was passed, the GOP moved to capitalize on public uncertainty about its cost and scope. Some Republicans spoke of repeal. Obama and congressional Democrats argued that voters would welcome the new benefits and reward their party for delivering on a promise.

But beneath all of this is the undeniable: that Obama will be remembered as the president who pulled off one of the most audacious legislative feats in nearly 40 years.

It was a monumental battle with unlikely characters—Roman Catholic bishops, "tea party" protesters, dying patients and an upstart Republican in Massachusetts. In the end, the saga vividly illustrated how individual actors can shape the course of history.

Those individuals emerged in the closing months of Obama's year-long march, from House Speaker Nancy Pelosi (D-Calif.), who would defy some of her closest allies to pass a bill; to Sen. Joseph I. Lieberman (I-Conn.), who would exert his leverage to force substantive changes; to Kennedy, who spent his dying days pressing for health-care reform; to Obama himself, who realized in early 2010 that to keep his presidency on track he would have to personally salvage his signature domestic initiative.

A rescue effort. That's what it came down to at the end for a president who one year earlier was newly inaugurated, full of hope, and full of confidence that this time was going to be different.

* * *

If there was a single operating principle for health-care reform in the early months of the Obama presidency, it was this: Don't do like the Clintons did.

Many in the White House, especially Emanuel, had lived through the failure of 1993–94, a debacle that cost Democrats control of both the House and Senate. The Obama team, determined not to repeat those mistakes, laid down a few basic rules:

- Do not write a bill. Members of Congress view that as their job and had balked when first lady Hillary Clinton delivered her blueprint to Capitol Hill.
- Do not emphasize the problems of the uninsured. Focus on the rising costs that worry middle-class voters and the corporate world.
- Move fast. Presidential honeymoons, and enthusiasm for large-scale initiatives, fade quickly.
- Neutralize the opposition. Find a way to deal with the industries and special interests that had crushed the Clinton effort.

So it was on March 5, 2009, that Obama welcomed to the White House a collection of 150 men and women who rarely, if ever, gather in one place together. Into the gold-toned East Room came Democratic and Republican lawmakers, leaders from organized labor and the American Medical Association, corporate executives, consumer advocates and officials from the U.S. Chamber of Commerce.

Most strikingly, the forum attracted many of the combatants who had made their reputations defeating "HillaryCare"—people such as W.J. "Billy" Tauzin, from the drug lobby, Karen Ignagni, representing insurers, and Chip Kahn, a hospital representative who had masterminded the iconic "Harry and Louise" ads for the insurance industry in the 1990s.

The irony was not lost on the participants, who had taken to calling themselves "strange bedfellows" in secret talks organized early on by Kennedy.

"We understand that we have to earn a seat at the table," said Ignagni, head of the trade group America's Health Insurance Plans. "I just wanted to get rid of the elephant in the room."

During the presidential transition, Obama surrogates had been making overtures to key players. Tauzin, head of the Pharmaceutical Research and Manufacturers of America (PhRMA), had quiet conversations with Thomas A. Daschle, a former senator who was slated to be Obama's health czar.

The strategy, as articulated by Emanuel, was to disarm—if not outright co-opt—potential opponents.

Temperamentally, the president and his chief of staff were polar opposites: Emanuel a hyperkinetic, profane creature of Washington to Obama's cool, detached, outsider persona. But the pair shared Chicago roots and a pragmatism not often found in partisan politics today.

From the outset, the two knew they would encounter industry resistance, but they also recognized they could not win an all-out war if the drug, hospital, physician and insurance lobbies combined forces against them. "Divide and conquer," Emanuel would say in staff meetings.

The administration's back-channel messages were part enticement, part threat. A new law that vastly expanded health insurance would translate into as many as 40 million additional customers—revenue the industry desperately wanted. Conversely, if they didn't join in the effort, they could expect harsh new regulations and steep cuts in government payments.

As chamber president Thomas J. Donohue put it that day in early March: "If you don't get in this game . . . you're on the menu."

Obama and Emanuel also understood that most Republicans would oppose them. But in the upbeat early days of the administration, they thought some amount of bipartisanship was possible. (At the time, it was also a necessity; Democrats did not have 60 reliable votes in the Senate to overcome filibusters.)

From a public relations standpoint, the televised forum was a coup. It showed Obama in command of the subject, in touch with average Americans' concerns and seemingly moving fast on an issue important to the public. Indeed, several Republicans made encouraging comments about the need to address flaws in the health-care system.

But offstage, the large-scale initiative had gotten off to a balky start.

Daschle, an Obama confidant who had written a book outlining a roadmap for reform, had withdrawn his Cabinet nomination a month earlier over his failure to pay $140,000 in back taxes. The episode cost the president not only his lead strategist, a man chosen for his ability to navigate the congressional maze, but also precious time.

Another absence—that of Kennedy—was felt even more acutely. He and Obama had forged a close relationship in the Senate, a bond cemented in late January 2008 when the elder statesman endorsed Obama in the presidential race.

In August 2008, three months after receiving a diagnosis of terminal brain cancer, Kennedy had made an emotional appearance at the Democratic National Convention, describing health-care reform as the "cause of my life."

But the two men had not seen each other since Obama's inauguration on Jan. 20, 2009, when Kennedy suffered a seizure at a luncheon in the Capitol. Since then, Kennedy, 77, had been convalescing in Florida. But his health was declining and no one knew whether he would be strong enough to attend the White House forum on March 5.

A few days before, he flew to Washington, and from a desk in his home rehearsed a short speech with his wife and closest aides.

It wasn't until late the night before that the White House learned Kennedy hoped to appear. Arrangements were made, just in case, and the next day, as the session wound down, Kennedy arrived at the White House and was secreted away in the Green Room. Word spread. A parade of administration officials, many of them former Kennedy staffers, others just admirers, dropped by. As Obama entered the room, Kennedy slowly rose to his feet in a sign of deference.

"Ted, we're gonna get this done," Obama said. He picked up his mentor's cane in one hand and used the other to guide the dying senator into the East Room to loud and sustained applause. Kennedy settled into a front-row seat as Obama said, "It is thrilling to see you here, Teddy."

Then it was Kennedy's turn. Gripping a microphone, he abandoned the script he had prepared. His remarks meandered. He repeated himself. He reached for his closing lines.

"I'm looking forward to being a foot soldier in this undertaking," he said in his baritone voice, in what would be one of his last public appearances. "And this time, we will not fail."

The applause began again, and for the moment, anyway, the 150 strange bedfellows were getting along.

* * *

"What are you in for?" Sen. Max Baucus (D-Mont.) asked the chief executives of five of the nation's largest pharmaceutical companies.

It was June 2, 2009, three months after the White House gathering, and all of the goodwill and civility had evaporated. The health-care debate had shifted from Kennedy's stirring words to the crass Washington subject of dollars and cents.

As chairman of the Finance Committee, Baucus was in charge of putting together the Senate health-care bill. He needed about $1 trillion to pay for the legislation, and there were only two places to find that kind of money—new revenue (from sources such as taxes and fees) or budget savings.

"Health reform will benefit you," he told the executives. "But you don't get those benefits for free."

The drug manufacturers, like other medical businesses, were poised to reap tens of millions of new customers in an expanded health-care system. The logical tradeoff, by Baucus's way of thinking, was for the industry to help offset the cost by accepting smaller federal reimbursements or paying a new fee to the government. What the industry gave up on one side of the ledger, Baucus argued, would be more than made up by these newly insured patients.

He wanted to squeeze $100 billion in savings out of the drug sector over the next 10 years, an eye-popping figure that temporarily silenced the men around the table. It was more than triple what they were considering. But Tauzin, a former congressman from Louisiana, didn't blink.

The companies were ready to contribute, he replied, but they didn't want Baucus simply to trim federal drug spending. They were offering big discounts on prescription medicines purchased through the Medicare program. The savings would accrue to senior citizens, not the government, Tauzin acknowledged, and the companies wanted credit for that.

"Senator, if you're willing to make that part of the discussion and it counts, we're willing to talk," he said.

Secret discussions between the industry, Baucus's aides and White House health czar Nancy-Ann DeParle had been underway throughout the spring. Each side had its reasons for being at the table—and a list of demands.

Obama needed the money, but more important, he wanted a few industry players on his side in what was certain to be a grueling and expensive battle. The industry, meanwhile, aimed to burnish its image, avoid onerous new regulations and have some degree of financial certainty.

Still, the executives were uncomfortable with Washington-style bartering. They were accustomed to hiring squadrons of lawyers to negotiate precisely worded contracts. This business was being done by the seat of the pants, big numbers tossed around with nothing on paper. And on most days, these men were rivals competing for market share, not partners in some political pact.

But Tauzin argued that the first industry group to cut a deal would fare the best. "It's an invitation you can't refuse," he would tell the corporate types.

In a show of good faith—or a reminder of its ability to shape public attitudes—the trade association was already airing television commercials loosely in support of an Obama-style overhaul.

Yet the president's hopes for speedy action on his centerpiece domestic issue were fading. Congress, mired in legislative minutiae, had made little progress, and the White House had been unable to finalize a single outside agreement. The pressure was on for a deal.

Slowly, the negotiators in the pharmaceutical talks closed in on a number: $80 billion over a decade. Some administration aides had expected a larger figure, but DeParle and White House Deputy Chief of Staff Jim Messina, who also had worked for Baucus, thought it would be better to lock in the smaller amount without a fight than risk a protracted brawl with no guarantee of money.

Even with the dollar amount resolved, the two sides were still far apart on the other details of an agreement, such as how to allocate the money and what relief the firms could expect on the regulatory front.

As the talks inched along in the days after the June 2 meeting, there was other discouraging news for the president.

At the start of the week of June 15, the independent Congressional Budget Office announced that the 10-year cost of the bill could easily reach $1.6 trillion, far more than what most lawmakers were willing to spend.

Two days later, the head of the office testified on Capitol Hill that the legislation would not meet Obama's central goal of reducing costs. It was an arcane discussion to be sure, but in the Byzantine world of lawmaking, it was a devastating blow.

On Wednesday, June 17, Baucus announced he was postponing action in his committee, another setback for the president, who had set summer as his deadline for passage.

Meanwhile, the haggling between Tauzin's team and the administration continued in private. White House negotiators pushed for penalties on manufacturers that did not provide the Medicare discounts. More significant, the two sides fought over which seniors would be eligible.

At one point, it appeared they had reached an accord. Then DeParle's cellphone rang. It was Emanuel, who understood so well the political clout of older voters. He had been studying polls showing that seniors needed a reason to support the health-care bill.

Push up the income threshold for the discounts, he instructed DeParle, worried that only the poorest of the elderly would qualify.

We're not slashing prices for wealthy seniors, the PhRMA lobbyists replied.

With that, the talks broke down.

On Thursday, June 18, half a dozen senior administration advisers gathered in Emanuel's West Wing office. If they had any chance of reviving the stalled health-care effort, they needed to generate some positive headlines. Their first choice was an agreement with the drugmakers, but that seemed stuck.

Some in the room blamed DeParle, who was hired in part because of her years of experience in the private sector.

She was annoyed with the White House number-crunchers, who couldn't seem to produce data to back up her theory that the drug companies were inflating prices.

They felt the momentum slipping away.

Emanuel, who had been privately griping that DeParle was not tough enough to close the deal, cut the meeting short.

"We're done fucking around," he barked. "Get it fucking done!"

* * *

The following day a deal was struck. In a conference call on the evening of Friday, June 19, the five pharmaceutical executives signed off on an agreement with Baucus and the Obama administration.

They were spurred in part by mounting concerns that the White House was preparing a public relations attack. Lobbyists for the drug companies were led to believe that if they did not reach a compromise, the president was preparing to target Big Pharma as the villain in the drama.

Once an accord was finalized, the White House PR machine spun in a different direction, portraying the deal as a victory for retirees. In a White House ceremony on Monday, Obama stood smiling beside the president of the seniors group AARP touting "the historic agreement to lower drug costs for seniors."

Not invited to pose at the photo opportunity were Tauzin and the chief executives. Tauzin wasn't upset; he understood that's the way it works in Washington. Some people the president wants to be pictured with, some people he doesn't.

But their contribution went well beyond the savings in the bill. During the year-long debate, the industry would spend about $150 million on pro-reform advertising, providing political cover to Democrats in tough reelection campaigns.

Equally important, the pharmaceutical deal became a template for others. In an arrangement similar to the drug accord, hospitals next agreed to forgo $155 billion in government reimbursements over 10 years.

Other heavyweights such as Wal-Mart, nurses and, to some degree, physicians spoke warmly about the president's initiative—statements coordinated and disseminated by the White House. Slowly, the Obama camp was removing potential adversaries from the battlefield.

The one major holdout was the insurance industry. But Emanuel, ever the political warrior, was content to pit the president against the unpopular industry. Regardless of whether insurers were the real cause of rising medical bills, polls showed that the public blamed them, and Obama frequently tapped into that anger to rally grass-roots support.

But the special-interest deals—and, later, the side bargains with individual lawmakers—were a double-edged sword for Obama. He had won the 2008 election as an agent of change, but the trading behind closed doors looked like the same old Washington.

Even allies questioned his actions.

Rep. Henry A. Waxman (D-Calif.), chairman of the House Energy and Commerce Committee, defiantly announced he was not bound by the agreements and, in fact, was drafting a bill that would extract a much larger contribution from drug manufacturers. His broadside, coupled with the lack of movement on Capitol Hill, alarmed the pharmaceutical executives.

Would Waxman prevail? How firm was the White House commitment? And what if Obama couldn't get a comprehensive bill passed?

On July 7, as congressional Democrats argued among themselves and Baucus searched in vain for Republican support for a bill, the pharmaceutical executives went to the White House for verification that their verbal agreement would hold.

AstraZeneca chief executive David Brennan spoke for the drugmakers, all seated in a row on one side of a table in the Roosevelt Room. Reading off a list of talking points they had prepared that morning, he reviewed the terms point by point.

Emanuel, seated across the table with Baucus, DeParle and Messina, listened for quite some time. Then, in his staccato shorthand, he reassured the executives that his side would not waver.

"You were first, I get it," he said. "We are in."

The executives worried about what might happen in the House as it considered its version of a bill, and they feared that lawmakers might still insert a change the industry vehemently opposed, a provision that would allow Americans to buy lower-priced drugs in countries such as Canada and "re-import" them into the United States.

"The House is the House," Emanuel said, with a dismissive wave of his hand.

Then more shorthand: "We're bound to this agreement and the Senate is bound to it."

Emanuel never made an explicit promise, but the group was heartened by his next comment.

"If health-care reform is done properly," he said, "the president doesn't think there will be a need for re-importation."

The strategy of engagement appeared to be working.

* * *

The deal-making of early July slipped into the gridlock of August.

Despite Obama's cajoling and badgering, despite the endorsements of PhRMA and AARP, Democrats in Congress could not agree on a bill.

In the House, Pelosi struggled to appease the disparate wings of her Democratic membership. They fought over taxes, Medicare payments, the cost of the legislation and whether to create a new government-sponsored insurance program known as a public option.

In the Senate, meanwhile, Baucus was struggling to craft a consensus bill in his Finance Committee. Convening daily sessions with a bipartisan group of senators dubbed the "Gang of Six," he had hinted for weeks that they were *so close* to achieving Obama's dream of bipartisanship. But the White House was tiring of the Kabuki theater.

As irritated as the Obama team was with its friends in Congress, Democratic lawmakers and loyalists were equally aggravated with the president. For weeks, he had refused to weigh in on intraparty disputes, particularly over the public option and tax treatment of high-priced insurance policies. His rambling performance during a prime-time news conference on health care only increased concern.

The White House team knew that time was its enemy, as the president's poll numbers showed soft spots and Republicans fanned growing unease about the legislation.

Early in the month, Emanuel gathered a small team to secretly begin drafting a White House bill. If Baucus didn't move soon, Emanuel wanted to be ready with a measure to send directly to the Senate floor, bypassing the committee. He calculated that the simple act of putting together a rival blueprint might be enough to jolt Baucus into action.

And Emanuel, fed up with a spate of news leaks, warned the aides in trademark fashion: "If this gets out, I'll fucking kill you."

On Capitol Hill, where recess periods are sacrosanct, lawmakers escaped Washington without casting a single vote on health-care legislation.

But the mood beyond the Beltway was ferocious. Conservative

talk show hosts and tea party activists helped organize protests against "ObamaCare." A proposal to pay for end-of-life counseling became "death panels" in the words of critics. Lawmakers were heckled and shouted down; the image of one congressman was hanged in effigy.

The president briefly hit the road, knocking down some of the more outrageous myths. But the damage had been done. Public opinion on health-care reform and Obama was turning sour.

Then came word that Kennedy, the benefactor who had persuaded the president to risk so much time and political capital on one issue, had died. Obama, looking to recharge after a grueling seven months in office, received the call while vacationing with his family on Martha's Vineyard.

On Aug. 29, as a steady rain fell, some 1,500 mourners filed into the Basilica of Our Lady of Perpetual Help in the Roxbury section of Boston. They were former presidents and prime ministers, Hollywood celebrities, sports stars and a busload of U.S. senators.

Many milling about under the twin spires that Saturday morning were the central characters in health-care fights past, present and yet to come, the very people Obama and Kennedy had hoped would make "health care for all" more than just a slogan. They included a raft of Democratic politicians such as Pelosi, Baucus and Senate Majority Leader Harry M. Reid (Nev.); Republican senators such as Orrin G. Hatch (Utah) and Olympia J. Snowe (Maine); White House aides; lobbyists; and Bill and Hillary Clinton; Podesta, who had watched Obama flop in Las Vegas in 2007; Daschle, who would have been the administration's health chief; and a woman named Martha Coakley, who aspired to replace Kennedy in the Senate.

Seated in the front row with his wife and vice president, Obama prepared to deliver his first eulogy as president. He did not intend to use it to make a pitch for the health-care legislation. He wanted to give a warm, personal speech, a proper Irish send-off for the Senate stalwart who had bestowed early legitimacy on his unlikely presidential candidacy.

Waiting for the Mass to begin, Obama draped his right arm over the back of the wooden pew and tilted his head toward Bill Clinton, seated behind him.

The two chatted for several minutes, seemingly oblivious to their surroundings and the myriad cameras aimed at them. Of all the whispered murmurings taking place in the prelude to Kennedy's funeral, the animated conversation between Obama and Clinton was surely the most closely watched.

But it was another brief exchange that carried greater political import that day—and beyond.

Standing at the edge of Obama's pew was a bearded man in crimson robes. Obama rose to his feet as Cardinal Sean O'Malley reached for his hand. O'Malley, the archbishop of Boston, welcomed the president and offered condolences. Then the highest-ranking Roman Catholic in ultra-Catholic Boston, in a private moment during this public gathering, delivered an unusually pointed message.

"The bishops are anxious to support health care," O'Malley said. "It's very important."

"But," the prelate added, still gripping Obama's hand, "we are very concerned that there not be public funding for abortion."

At the time, it might have seemed little more than a discordant note at a memorial service. But O'Malley's words foreshadowed the arduous struggle about to unfold once everyone was back in Washington—and the contentious issue that would almost derail Obama's quest to make health-care history.

CHAPTER 2

The House of Pelosi: Deals and Betrayals

Early on the morning of Nov. 2, 2009, Nancy Pelosi settled into the chair behind her desk at the U.S. Capitol. The view from her second-floor office is breathtaking—down the sloping lawn of the Capitol to the National Mall all the way to the Washington Monument.

But on that Monday, her gaze was trained on the list of names placed beside a bowl of fresh flowers. It was time for Pelosi to do what she does as well as any modern-day House speaker: lock in votes one deal at a time.

The raw numbers favored Pelosi—there were 256 Democrats in the House, and she would gain two more in special elections the next day. All she needed were 218 votes to seal the biggest legislative accomplishment of her career by passing comprehensive health-care reform, a feat that had eluded every other House speaker who had tried.

Yet even 218 posed a challenge. The Democrats had splintered into disparate factions, and Pelosi had spent much of the fall slogging through seemingly endless negotiations, trying to assemble even a fragile coalition. Controlling her caucus and rounding up stragglers now came down to one critical week. With the Veterans Day recess approaching, Pelosi calculated that she had six days, maybe seven, to secure votes for President Obama's proposal before lawmakers left for the holiday. She started dialing.

She tracked down Rep. Jim Cooper (D-Tenn.) in a Tennessee airport, returning to Washington for the final week. Cooper was a long shot—he helped defeat the Clinton initiative in 1994.

"I'm not first on her list," he said wryly the next day. Still, Pelosi had to try; she needed votes.

" 'The store is open,' " Cooper recalled Pelosi telling him. " 'We're crafting the manager's amendment. Now is the time to get in your provisions.' "

She reached 50 or so Democrats that day, cataloguing their wants and gripes, tucking into a folder her notes from each conversation.

It was a skill she had mastered at an early age. Pelosi was just 8 years old when her father, Tommy D'Alesandro, a legendary mayor of Baltimore, taught her to record the requests of each constituent in an index-card box known as the "favor file."

Now at age 69, Pelosi had her own constituents—258 Democratic lawmakers, each with a favor to ask. Many, like Cooper, remained uncertain. By Pelosi's math, she had more than 200 solid commitments but was still a dozen or so votes short.

With each passing day, she called in chits and piled up promises. She said she would raise the limit on a tax on the wealthy in the measure and picked up two votes. She agreed to an insurance change that would allow children through age 26 to stay on a parent's policy, ensuring another vote.

Three more for the favor file.

She promised to improve the Indian Health Service and spend more money on anti-rejection drugs for transplant patients. She vowed to trim a medical-devices tax and close a possible loophole that would let paper companies claim a tax break on a by-product known as "black liquor."

The favor file grew. The tally of "yes" votes inched closer to 218.

The Pelosi touch wasn't perfect. When she spotted Rep. Walt Minnick in the hall, she made her pitch. But the lone Democrat from Idaho politely reminded the speaker he had been a "no" for some time.

Hispanic lawmakers threatened to bolt over the treatment of illegal immigrants in the Senate's legislation. Pelosi sent them to the White House, where Obama quelled the rebellion.

Pelosi had other uprisings to contend with. Most worrisome was an incendiary issue that had long bedeviled the Democratic Party, an issue Pelosi, the first female speaker of the House, had hoped would be resolved before the vote.

* * *

For nearly 40 years, Democrats had grappled with the crosscurrents of the abortion issue. Few members embodied those tensions more than Pelosi. A practicing Catholic, she bucked church leadership by becoming a stalwart defender of the right to choose. In the House, some of Pelosi's most loyal support came from women lawmakers who shared her views.

The first rumblings surfaced over the summer. In committee debate, Democratic Rep. Bart Stupak, a stubborn former Michigan cop, tried to insert strict new abortion limits in the bill. He pushed an amendment that would prohibit coverage for the procedure in any health plan that included individuals receiving government subsidies. Stupak's opponents said it would make it impossible for any woman to purchase the coverage, even with her own money.

After the amendment was defeated in committee, Boston's Catholic archbishop weighed in directly with Obama at Kennedy's funeral in August. A few weeks later, in a joint address to Congress, the president declared: "Under our plan, no federal dollars will be used to fund abortions."

At that point, Obama and Pelosi believed the issue had been put to rest. Her committee chairmen had crafted language that she thought satisfied both sides. It would allow health plans to offer abortion coverage as long as private and public money were kept separate.

But the bishops and Stupak were not mollified. By that first week in November, as Pelosi made her final push for 218, they pressed anew for the more restrictive approach.

The bishops sent a dispatch marked "urgent" to every U.S. parish advocating defeat of the bill if it did not include Stupak's amendment. They distributed fliers picturing a pregnant woman and the message: "Abortion is not health care, because killing is not healing."

They tapped Raymond Flynn, a former U.S. ambassador to the Vatican, to record a phone message decrying the measure, while a dozen bishops interceded with lawmakers.

Pelosi was accustomed to battling the church, but she also understood the clout the bishops carried with wavering Catholic lawmakers. A handful of Pelosi's deputies—senior Democrats she trusted—tried going around Stupak. While he was attending a funeral in Michigan, they floated another compromise with a junior member of the antiabortion contingent. If they could peel off just a few members, Pelosi would have her 218 votes, and Stupak would be rendered irrelevant.

Stupak was incensed. "They were trying to cut separate deals to break up our coalition," he said later.

On Friday, Nov. 6, on his return to Washington, Stupak organized a meeting of the antiabortion coalition. More than a dozen lawmakers, along with the bishops' representatives, gathered in a hearing room of the Rayburn House Office Building. Stupak called in from Chicago's O'Hare International Airport.

"We must stay united," he implored over his cellphone. "Let's not fold; let's hold firm to the Stupak language."

Stupak's coalition remained united. The end run wasn't going to work, and Pelosi's hope for a quick resolution vanished. It was time for the speaker, who had left the abortion negotiations to her lieutenants, to take on the problem herself.

She invited the Democratic women in the House to her conference room. Seated at the head of the long, polished wood table, she pleaded for them not to let a "sidebar issue" crush what she called a historic opportunity to improve the lives of millions of women who lacked adequate medical care.

"The abortion issue should never have been a part of this," Pelosi told her political sisters. "The more you talk about something other than what the bill does, it's a victory for those who want to defeat the bill. So don't take the bait."

The session touched on hardheaded calculations and deeply personal matters. The women debated when life begins and what the polls meant.

"We can talk about different language, but we are not going to agree to further restrictions on a woman's right to choose," warned Rep. Diana DeGette (D-Colo.), co-chairman of the Congressional Pro-Choice Caucus.

"I understand what women are going through across this country," countered Rep. Kathy Dahlkemper (D-Pa.), one of only two lawmakers in the room who opposed abortion rights. She made an oblique reference to her experience as a young, unwed mother. Having an abortion might have been "the easier route," she said. "But then my son and grandchild would not be here today."

Rep. Marcy Kaptur (D-Ohio), feeling like the only other "radish in a green salad," praised Dahlkemper. "That was very courageous to speak out with such feeling," she said to dead silence. "Of course, what underlies this are very serious moral and theological disagreements about when life begins."

As she spoke, a collective groan went out, cutting her off midthought. Kaptur felt very alone, and more determined than ever not to cave on a moral issue about which she felt so strongly.

The women were at a stalemate—and Pelosi had no more than 36 hours before the scheduled vote.

"We're standing on the brink of doing something great," she said. "I'm not letting anything stand in the way of that."

* * *

The speaker's suite—a warren of connecting offices and conference rooms down a long, narrow passageway off the Capitol Rotunda—enables Pelosi to hold several meetings simultaneously. By late afternoon Friday, one day before the vote, she was shuttling, cellphone in hand, from room to room.

In one, she talked parliamentary strategy. In another, she conferred with a small group of the most senior women in the House. Stupak had boasted that he controlled 40 Democratic votes. Pelosi's count showed that fewer than six actually hung on the outcome of the abortion dispute—but she needed nearly every one.

"We have two options," she told the women. "Do something that allows us to get agreement with the bishops, or I have to pull the bill."

Because of the rules of the House, Pelosi would need to survive three floor votes: the vote on the health-care legislation, plus two procedural challenges. Any one of the three could spell defeat for the measure. Pelosi feared that Republicans could beat her on a procedural motion by inserting a "poison pill," legislative language that exploited the Democratic divisions over abortion and immigration. Combining the two issues was "an explosive situation for us," she said.

She juggled phone calls from allies at Planned Parenthood, and Catholic leaders such as Cardinal Theodore E. McCarrick in Rome and Cardinal Francis George, president of the U.S. Conference of Catholic Bishops. She was caught in the middle, vowing to find a compromise.

"I want to get this done," one lawmaker heard Pelosi tell George. "I'm going into a meeting to try to do exactly what it is we all want to do, and that is pass a health-care bill."

As she finished the call, Pelosi returned to the conference room where that morning she had appealed to her female colleagues. After months of keeping her distance, the speaker now sat face to face with the men who stood in her way: the lobbyists for the Catholic bishops and Stupak.

"Explain to me what is the problem," she said. "I want to hear this myself. Why do you believe we haven't addressed the question of no federal dollars being used to pay for abortion?"

From across the table, several chairs down, came the gravelly voice of a man who suddenly tipped the balance of power in Washington. In a city where individuals can exert outsize influence, Richard Doerflinger, one of the most ardent leaders in the Catholic Church's antiabortion movement, was doing just that.

Segregating tax money from private insurance payments was no more than a "clever accounting maneuver," he said. He passed out a memo detailing the bishops' objections.

"I don't care what accounting gimmick you come up with," he said, in typical blunt fashion.

As Stupak sat silent, Doerflinger recited a history of federal abortion regulations. A few of Pelosi's allies parried with Doerflinger. What he was demanding went beyond existing law, they said.

The session stretched on for nearly three hours. Doerflinger insisted that the Stupak amendment was their "bottom line."

Pelosi and others pressed Stupak on how many votes he controlled.

Twelve or 15, he replied.

They wanted names.

"I'm not gonna tell you," he said.

"Where do you have Lipinski?" they asked, referring to one undecided lawmaker, Rep. Daniel Lipinski (D-Ill.).

"He's a 'no,'" Stupak said. "If you give me a vote on my amendment, I think he'll be a 'yes.'" Stupak even claimed he could deliver a Republican: Rep. Anh "Joseph" Cao (La.).

Stupak and Doerflinger wouldn't budge. Pelosi was nearly out of time. A historic health-care vote was within her grasp, and she was not about to be outmaneuvered. In a cold calculation to regain the power she had wielded so effectively all week, she decided to make the ultimate deal.

* * *

Shortly after 8 p.m., as Stupak and the Catholic lobbyists drifted out of the speaker's suite, Pelosi summoned her closest friends and colleagues for what would be the most trying meeting of a long and draining week.

The Democrats filed into the conference room: Majority Leader Steny H. Hoyer (Md.) and DeGette, who raced from the House gym. Rep. Rosa DeLauro (Conn.), a Catholic who had tried to work out an earlier compromise, and Rep. George Miller (Calif.), perhaps Pelosi's most trusted ally. Rep. Henry A. Waxman (Calif.), who had written much of the bill, and Rep. Louise M. Slaughter (N.Y.), who had climbed the leadership ladder with Pelosi since their arrival in Congress in 1987.

At age 80, Slaughter headed the House Rules Committee, giving her tremendous control over when and how votes would take place, and making her one of the nation's most powerful politicians—though she was far from nationally known.

For Slaughter, more than many, the abortion issue was also intensely personal. As a young woman in Kentucky, she had helped protect a friend's secret: a risky, illegal abortion. Ever since, she had fought to keep the procedure legal, in the early years marching through the streets and later leveraging her clout in Congress.

Since 2 p.m., Slaughter's committee had been preparing the rules for the next day's vote, normally a routine step for legislation headed to the House floor. But, knowing that the bill's fate rested on Pelosi's negotiations with the bishops, Slaughter had stalled for hours.

Once Pelosi's team was gathered around her at the head of the table, she recapped the session with Stupak and the bishops. "I don't know what to do," she said. "They want their amendment."

In truth, she knew what she had to do. But it was difficult to break the news to this group, particularly the women who felt a deep bond with her. She let several talk, some imploring her for more time.

Then she displayed her tally sheets. "I don't have the votes for final passage," Pelosi said.

"I looked at the list, and she was right," DeGette observed later.

Slowly, each person in the room came to the realization that Pelosi was considering embedding Stupak's tough, new abortion limits into the broader health-care legislation. A vote for the bill would be a vote for the very abortion restrictions they so loathed.

The women were furious. They had given enough. Voices were raised, and DeLauro and Miller clashed in a heated exchange. Two participants said Pelosi had tears in her eyes.

"It was infuriating to think: Here we have the first female speaker of the House, strongly pro-choice. We have 190 members in the Pro-Choice Caucus, and we're being held hostage by the bishops," DeGette said later.

Slaughter, seething, lamented "all the women we were just throwing under the bus" with the Stupak provision, adding, "It was a betrayal of all the women that had fought for this for so long."

Pelosi tried reassurance, saying this wasn't the final step. There would be opportunities to change the abortion language later in the process.

"It wasn't as if this was making policy for the country," she said. "It was about passing a bill to take us to the next step."

That may be, the women countered, but it was a risk. And they weren't going to make it easy for Stupak. They wanted a roll-call vote so that every lawmaker would be on record for or against an amendment that they said "turned back the clock" on women's rights.

Close to 11 p.m., the women angrily fled the suite, storming past a phalanx of reporters.

On the third floor, Stupak, Doerflinger and their allies swept into the cramped Rules Committee room to formally present the abortion amendment.

Slaughter, even though she was the committee chairman, headed for her office adjacent to the hearing room, refusing to preside over the panel's work. She would not challenge her dear friend Pelosi's decision, but she also would not participate in passing a measure she so viscerally opposed.

Instead, she pulled a yellow chair up to a bank of television screens in the office. The two other Democratic women on the committee—Doris Matsui of California and Chellie Pingree of Maine—left the hearing room and joined her.

Next door, Dahlkemper spoke in favor of Stupak's amendment, again citing her experiences as an unwed mother. The remaining committee Democrats, reluctantly following Pelosi's instructions, could do little more than make dark references to back-alley procedures and coat hangers.

When it came time for the committee to approve the rules for the next day's floor debate, Slaughter, Matsui and Pingree didn't budge from the adjacent office. They refused to vote, instead watching it all unfold on C-SPAN.

Pelosi did not wait for the Rules Committee vote. She was headed home when the roll was called. After a week of horse-trading and a final concession that had infuriated her close friends and political allies, she now knew how the drama would end: The next day, when the full House took up the bill, she would have her votes.

Nancy Pelosi would go down in history as the speaker who passed the most sprawling piece of health-care legislation in generations. She would be the one who had done it.

CHAPTER 3

The Power of One:
Lieberman Blocks the Way

On the second Sunday in November, President Obama made a rare weekend appearance in the Rose Garden to praise the House for its vote.

"For years we've been told that this couldn't be done," he marveled. "But last night, the House proved differently."

The final vote—220 to 215—suggested to some a fragile victory for the president. But viewed another way, the fact that the bill passed at all underscored the power of Pelosi, who had cajoled and bartered for those 220 votes.

The power of one person: That was what Pelosi had proven shapes legislation in Washington. But even as Obama spoke, that power was shifting and being redefined.

A few blocks from the White House, Sen. Joseph I. Lieberman (I-Conn.) was appearing on *Fox News Sunday*. "I will not allow this bill to come to a final vote," he said. And in the flash of a sound bite, the battle over health-care reform moved to the Senate, and the power of one took on an entirely different cast.

In the House, Pelosi exerted singular authority. She, and she alone, had the ability to grant favors, approve changes and extract painful concessions. But in the Senate, the balance of power on the issue resided with a few centrists such as Lieberman, each of whom knew that 60 votes would be needed to overcome filibusters and pass a bill.

They also knew that Majority Leader Harry M. Reid (D-Nev.) needed all 58 Democrats and the Senate's two independents to reach the magical 60. With not a vote to spare, that meant any wavering senator would have to be dealt with.

And Lieberman, who was one of those two independents—and who had earned a reputation as a great waverer—had just made clear: He was ready to be dealt with.

* * *

Of the myriad adjectives Democrats used to describe Lieberman, "wavering" was one of the more polite ones.

For decades he had been one of them, even running on the Democratic ticket in 2000 as Al Gore's vice presidential pick. Six years later, in his Senate reelection campaign, Lieberman lost the Democratic primary, ran as an independent and won.

By 2008, when he endorsed Republican Sen. John McCain (Ariz.) over Obama in the presidential race, Democrats considered his betrayal complete. Yet Lieberman caucused with Senate Democrats, and Reid—inexplicably to some—had allowed him to keep a committee chairmanship.

During moments of reflection, Lieberman, a devout Jew, would say he did not enjoy being an outcast, especially in the clubby Senate. But he viewed each party break as a principled move and, as he became a more seasoned Washington player, a fresh opportunity to leverage influence.

Five weeks after his Fox appearance, Lieberman returned to the Sunday talk-show circuit.

"We've got to stop adding to the bill," he said on *Face the Nation*. "We've got to start subtracting some controversial things."

It was Dec. 13, less than two weeks before Congress would break for the Christmas holidays. Although the Senate debate had dragged on for two full weeks already, Reid still did not have 60 votes.

His troops were stuck on what role the government should play in a revamped health-care system. Liberals were wedded to the awkwardly named "public option," a proposal to create a voluntary government-sponsored insurance program that they said would hold in check private insurers.

But Lieberman and other centrists refused to support the public option, saying it was just a back-door path to an eventual government takeover of the entire system.

Scrambling to break the impasse before the recess, Reid used a classic Washington maneuver: a bit of PR sleight of hand. Mid-week, the Democratic leader tantalized reporters with word of a major breakthrough. He declined to discuss the details, but said a tentative accord had been struck to appease his party's liberal wing. In place of a public insurance program, Reid would insert a provision allowing people between the ages of 55 and 65 to "buy in" to the Medicare program.

The idea, promoted by former Vermont governor Howard Dean, a Democrat, was in some ways even more attractive to progressives than the public option. Opening up Medicare to millions of pre-retirees would significantly expand the government's role in the health-care system.

Reid and the White House believed they had Lieberman cornered; as Gore's running mate, he had endorsed extending Medicare to young retirees and spoke favorably of the idea again in September in a videotaped interview with a newspaper. When an aide caught wind of the possible deal, he sent a frantic BlackBerry message to Lieberman, who was attending a friend's farewell dinner at the exclusive Alibi Club in Washington.

In truth, the Senate negotiators had not promised to vote for the proposed change, but merely to pursue it as an alternative. Still, Lieberman knew how Washington worked; he could feel the ground shifting. In a city where perception often becomes reality, he feared that once the media concluded the logjam had been broken, it would become a fait accompli.

"I was concerned about the way this was being handled in the press," Lieberman said later. "This is politics, nothing evil about it. But Harry and Chuck were really building up a kind of public mood that we basically had an agreement, that they had the 60 votes, and it was done," he added, referring to Reid and Sen. Charles E. Schumer (D-N.Y.).

Sipping freshly brewed espresso in his office, Lieberman explained his next moves.

By his calculation, Reid and Obama were a long way from lining up a single Republican vote. That meant they needed him more than ever.

"They made the decision they've got to get me," he said. "I'm not going to be unreasonable, but I've been clear about what I don't want."

On Dec. 10, he wrote his concerns in a private letter to Reid.

"Regarding the 'Medicare buy-in' proposal, the more I learn about it, the less I like it," he wrote. True, he had supported the idea in the past, "but that was a very different time. The federal government had a surplus, Medicare wasn't facing imminent bankruptcy, and there wasn't a health-care reform bill that created a vast new system of subsidies and tax credits and exchanges."

When the letter failed to stop Reid's move, Lieberman decided to use another tool of savvy Washington politicians: He went on television.

The Medicare expansion suffered "some of the same infirmities that the public option did," he said on CBS. It was just more government meddling that the nation couldn't afford.

The way things stood, Lieberman said, he was prepared to filibuster Obama's health-care overhaul. He listed his demands. "No public option," he said. "No Medicare buy-in."

Within moments, Reid frantically began phoning aides, White House officials and other senators. By the time Lieberman drove from the television studio downtown to his Georgetown home, the majority leader was calling him.

Even more than on the final vote, Reid needed Lieberman's support on a series of procedural tests. He asked Lieberman to simply help him move the bill along. If the final version was unacceptable, Reid urged, go ahead and vote no. But help me get past these parliamentary hurdles, he implored.

"I don't want to vote against the bill, Harry," Lieberman replied. "I want to vote for the bill." But he knew that under the rules of the Senate, his greatest leverage came on the procedural votes where 60 senators were needed to overcome a filibuster.

"The only option I have" is to block the legislation, he said.

The health-care battle had taken a political toll on Reid, a soft-spoken former boxer and gambling commissioner who started each day at dawn by reading a Bible passage. Critics—and even many Democratic allies—blamed him for allowing the Senate negotiations to drag on from early June well past Thanksgiving. Back home, his reelection prospects looked bleak.

Yet Reid had managed to hold his fractious caucus together. To get this far, he had promised $300 million in extra Medicaid money to Sen. Mary Landrieu (D-La.), in a deal dubbed the "Louisiana Purchase," and had agreed to trim a new tax on medical device manufacturers to woo several Midwestern senators.

"There's a hundred senators here, and I don't know if there is a senator that doesn't have something in this bill that was important to them. And if they don't have something in it important to them, then it doesn't speak well of them," he said.

But now Reid was agitated. He knew there was more negotiating to come, but he thought Lieberman would be satisfied after the government-sponsored public option was removed from the bill.

"This is over," Reid said in an urgent phone call to Rahm Emanuel, the White House chief of staff.

"Harry, calm down," Emanuel replied, as he drove his son home from bar mitzvah class. "I'll be over to your office soon."

The phone calls continued, from the Capitol to Lieberman's home to Emanuel's speeding car. Reid asked colleagues to try to convince Lieberman, but they were unsuccessful. Finally, he called Lieberman again: Come to a meeting in my office this afternoon.

* * *

Before Lieberman arrived, Emanuel, other White House aides and several senators gathered in the office tucked in a corner of the Capitol near the Senate chamber.

"Everyone was furious, furious," said one lawmaker in the room. "We're not going to meet Joe Lieberman's demands."

At best, Reid had 58 "yes" votes, two shy of what he needed— and he had yet to begin serious negotiations with the Senate's other great waverer, Ben Nelson (Neb.).

Reid was subdued, but visibly upset.

"Lieberman just wasn't honest with me," he said. "I can't believe he did this."

Some in the room spoke of going back to the bargaining table with Republican Sen. Olympia J. Snowe (Maine); others said, "Screw it, we may not have a bill."

As they blew off steam, Kate Leone, Reid's top health adviser, spoke up.

"How can you let all this go down the drain?" she said. "This is a good bill. As infuriating as this is, you can't let your anger at Senator Lieberman undo all this work."

Grudgingly, they agreed to cut a deal with Lieberman—but it would be the last.

"Okay, let's get right to it," Reid said when Lieberman arrived. "We need your vote. I want to know clearly what you want."

Lieberman reiterated his demands: no public option, no Medicare expansion. Other minor items were on his list, but those were the two issues on which he would not compromise.

"I understand your position," Reid said. "I'm not happy about it, but I've got to deal with it." The public option was already gone, and he would drop the Medicare buy-in.

In return, they extracted a pledge from Lieberman: This was it. No more reasons to vote against the bill.

They had a deal.

Still, Reid's allies fumed, whispering to reporters that Lieberman had double-crossed them.

"It's all coming down to one guy who's prepared to vote against the interests of children and families in Connecticut who need health-care reform," one Reid aide told the newspaper *Roll Call*, speaking on the condition of anonymity.

The next morning, the phone lines, Internet and cable television crackled with speculation. Activists on the left were angry over the notion that a turncoat like Lieberman held such sway. They questioned his motives, saying he was a shill for his home-state insurance industry. His Connecticut colleague, Democratic Rep. Rosa DeLauro, urged his recall. The liberal grass-roots group MoveOn.org quickly spearheaded a fundraising drive against him.

In the anteroom to Lieberman's Capitol Hill office suite, two young aides scrambled to answer telephones. The senator had catapulted into the health-care headlines, and it seemed that nearly everyone had an opinion on his behavior.

"He has doctors that advise him," said one staffer in response to a caller's question about how Lieberman got his information.

"He is in favor of tort reform," said another, fielding a call from a Republican constituent.

"Well, he's concerned about what it means for current Medicare beneficiaries," said the first, explaining the senator's comments on CBS.

In the hall outside, a TV crew waited for a shot of the lawmaker causing all the fuss. Meanwhile, liberal bloggers had begun a petition drive urging the Susan G. Komen for the Cure cancer foundation to dump Lieberman's wife, Hadassah, as its "global ambassador" because her husband "is pledging to kill health-care reform while millions go untreated."

"That goes over the line," Lieberman said in his private office. "There's no limit. What happens here is you take a position on an issue, and if they can't convince you to change your position, they try to intimidate you and attack your wife and so forth."

As the clock approached 5 p.m., the crowd of reporters staking out Lieberman's office swelled. They hoped to catch him on his way to a 5:30 meeting of Senate Democrats.

By 5:35, he emerged, a gaggle of aides serving as human shields. The scrum squeezed into an elevator and rode to the basement, where more reporters waited to cram into a subway car with the pack for the quick shuttle to the Capitol.

"Do you have a deal?" one hollered.

"Will you support the bill?" asked another.

As Lieberman stepped off the subway, more reporters joined the chase, the tangle of flying arms, cameras and microphones almost knocking over another senator.

By the time Lieberman entered the Lyndon B. Johnson Room, 50 paces off the Senate floor, most of the seats were filled. "Joe's here, now we can begin," one senator teased.

Reid faced a rebellion. Many of his rank-and-file members loathed the idea of ceding to Lieberman.

"I understand you're angry," Reid said. "I'm angry. But I just want to talk to you a little bit about what he's meant to the caucus this year."

Reid reminded them of the big votes of 2009—and the mathematical realities of Senate life.

Economic recovery package? Sixty votes, "and Joe was one of them," Reid said.

Children's health insurance? Sixty again.

Down the list he went.

"I know you're upset with him, but look what he's helped us do," the majority leader concluded. "We need him to make 60 votes on this."

Lieberman inched forward in his seat to speak, but others moved faster. Don't let one senator hold us hostage, someone growled. Maybe we need to change the rules on committee chairmanships, another suggested in a not-so-subtly veiled threat.

Finally, Paul Kirk, the man temporarily filling the seat of the late senator Edward M. Kennedy (D-Mass.), spoke. He said that Kennedy, the great champion of health-care reform, "knew when to fight and he knew when to close the deal," according to notes of the session. "While Teddy might have wanted a public option, at this moment he would say: This is a great achievement, let's get it done."

Lieberman stayed quiet, but the next day, at the White House, he decided to address his angry colleagues.

"This has been a difficult couple weeks for me because of the separation I've felt from people in the caucus," he said. "I know people are upset with me."

He took his time, highlighting what he liked in the bill, complimenting Reid and others on their work. But he also reminded them of the particular power each held.

"Every one of us is necessary to get to 60," he said. Others had said that having 60 senators in the caucus was both a blessing and a curse.

"It's really much more of a blessing, because we have the ability to work this out within this caucus," he said. "Just think where we'd be today in our quest for health-care reform if we had 55 or 57 or even 59."

* * *

With Lieberman finally on board, Reid had one more waverer to court. It took three more days—and promises of Medicaid money for Nebraska and changes to the abortion-funding restrictions—but just before 11 p.m. on Friday, Dec. 18, Reid locked in Nelson.

On Dec. 24, the Senate convened its first Christmas Eve session since 1895. In the frigid, early morning darkness, lawmakers filtered into the Capitol, many sporting snow boots and holiday ties.

After months of closed-door negotiations and 25 days of acrimonious floor debate, the outcome finally was assured. Democrats had their 60 votes.

The senators took their seats at compact, wooden desks for the roll call. When his turn came, Sen. Robert C. Byrd (D-W.Va.), 92 and in a wheelchair, thrust a pointed finger in the air.

"This is for my friend Ted Kennedy," he said in a quavering voice. "Aye!"

In the balcony above, Vicki Kennedy brushed away a tear. Her husband had fought for decades for this moment, and after the 60-to-39 vote, senators enveloped her in hugs.

"I voted twice," said Sen. John F. Kerry, who had served as the junior Democrat from Massachusetts for 24 years. "Once for me and once for Teddy."

As others raced to catch flights home, Sen. Christopher J. Dodd (D-Conn.) drove across the Potomac River to Arlington National Cemetery. There beside Kennedy's grave, marked by a plain white cross and flat marble footstone, he took a private moment to savor the victory.

There was still work to be done. They would have to resolve differences between the House and Senate versions of the legislation. But Democrats now felt certain that the goal of health-care reform—a quest that had eluded presidents for six decades, a quest that Kennedy called "the cause of my life"—seemed on the verge of becoming a reality.

CHAPTER 4

The Rescue: Obama's Last Chance

It was the Barack Obama that the American public rarely sees—irritated and wondering if he had arrived at the moment of defeat.

Shortly after 6 p.m. on Jan. 19, 2010, with a political crisis about to explode, the president summoned the two top Democrats in Congress to the Oval Office for a strategy session.

House Speaker Pelosi sat alongside Senate Majority Leader Reid, the tension in the room acute.

Obama wasn't waiting for the polls to close in Massachusetts at 8 that evening. Despite his last-ditch trip to Boston two days earlier, he knew that his Democratic Party was about to suffer an embarrassing loss. In the bitterest of ironies, the Senate seat held for nearly 47 years by Ted Kennedy was about to fall into Republican hands.

Now the president was asking members of his assembled brain trust: What were they going to do?

Although they shared Obama's desire to vastly expand the nation's health-care system, they were divided over how to salvage his policy proposal.

Mathematically, Scott Brown's impending victory would deny Democrats a filibuster-proof majority in the Senate. With only 59 votes loosely under his control, Reid wanted the House to adopt the version of the health-care bill that had barely squeaked through the Senate on Christmas Eve.

No way, Pelosi said.

"The Senate bill is a non-starter," she said. "I can't sell that to my members."

Pelosi lectured the others about the political realities of the House: Her Democratic troops did not trust the Senate, and she would face a mutiny if she asked them to do what Reid was suggesting.

They talked over each other, round and round, repeating the arguments Obama had heard for weeks.

"Let me finish," he broke in at one point.

"I understand that, Nancy," he snapped at another. "What's your solution?"

This was not how the president had envisioned things. He was just one day away from celebrating his first year in office. By now, he was to have signed into law the broadest piece of social policy legislation since President Lyndon B. Johnson's Great Society.

Instead, he was confronting the very real prospect of failure on an equally grand scale. The power of one person in Washington: On Jan. 19, that person seemed to be Scott Brown. But, really, it was now down to Obama. If he found a way to succeed, he would have his legislation. If not?

There went health-care reform.

There went history.

* * *

Panic. Despair. Back-stabbing. Recriminations. Calibrations and recalibrations.

From the evening hours of Jan. 19 through the next two months, Washington descended into full soap-opera mode.

As Pelosi and Reid left the White House that night, the administration was coming to the conclusion that its fatal mistake had been giving up so much control to Congress. Although the strategy was intended to correct for the mistakes President Bill Clinton made in 1993 when his wife's task force wrote a health-care bill in secret, the Obama White House belatedly realized that the months of delay, closed-door negotiations and special deals had tarnished the effort and a president who won office by promising to change the way Washington operates.

And so came the first attempt at a retooled strategy: a commander in chief back in charge. Obama would still need Pelosi and Reid to deliver votes, but this time the White House intended to steer more aggressively.

"In 2010, the president has to look like he is leading the process," communications director Dan Pfeiffer said in a meeting with the president and senior staffers. The goal is to "change the narrative" from the deal-making on Capitol Hill to "Obama finally taking charge of health reform."

On Jan. 29, Obama traveled to Baltimore for a rare appearance with House Republicans. The televised give-and-take showed him at his best, and it gave a psychological boost to his White House team, including his chief of staff, Rahm Emanuel, who proposed that Obama hold a bipartisan summit, much like the successful summit on welfare reform that Clinton had held in 1995.

Obama, who felt particularly stung by critics who said that he had broken his pledge to air the health-care debate on television, immediately embraced the summit concept. It would be a chance to reset the effort, display his willingness to accept Republicans' ideas, and claim—albeit more for show than substance—that he was crafting a "new" bill that was not sullied by the deals struck in Congress.

Privately, some of his key aides had doubts, such as health-care adviser Nancy-Ann DeParle and legislative liaison Phil Schiliro. They felt that they had tried for nearly a year to reach out to a handful of Republicans, with no success. Why give the GOP another opportunity to delay?

But Obama viewed the summit as a fresh chance to sell the public on his vision and highlight what he considered to be shortcomings in the Republican proposals. At a meeting in the Roosevelt Room a few hours after returning from Baltimore, he ridiculed health-care legislation sponsored by House Minority Leader John A. Boehner (R-Ohio).

"Covering 3 million people is not our goal," Obama reminded aides.

Emanuel, who served in the Clinton White House, raised the prospect of scaling back the bill, a theme he had struck several times over the previous year. As the architect of many of the small-bore initiatives in the Clinton era, Emanuel had periodically argued that it was "better to get points on the scoreboard" with a modest legislative success than to have nothing.

After the defeat in Massachusetts, he again asked aides to run the numbers on smaller-scale alternatives—as a fallback, at least. Most of the scenarios envisioned spending $150 billion to $500 billion over a decade and would focus on coverage for young adults or families with young children.

Obama considered what Emanuel was saying. For days, he had been hearing Pelosi's warnings that she could not round up the votes for the Senate bill. The speaker was one of the most skilled vote-counters in history; her assessment carried weight.

But Obama knew she was one of history's most skilled vote-getters as well. More than anyone else, in fact, she had been the reason the House had passed its health-care bill back in November. If Pelosi now said she might not be able to deliver a second time, Obama realized Emanuel's default plan could be the only option.

"Maybe we just can't get there," the president acknowledged. But let's at least try, he told his advisers.

"We're so close," he said. Bills have passed the House and Senate. "We're right there. Even if we are within the realm of possibility, we should go for it."

* * *

If Obama was beginning to reassert control behind the scenes, the message was more muddled in public. Although he continued to say he was determined to see lawmakers pass the legislation, he offered scant ideas for how they might do so.

On Capitol Hill, where fears of an electoral wipeout in the November midterm elections were coursing through the Democratic ranks because of the upset in Massachusetts, lawmakers grumbled that Obama was still leaving the hard work to them.

The president decided to meet them halfway—literally.

On Feb. 3, his limousine made the short ride down Pennsylvania Avenue to the Newseum, a few blocks from the Capitol. In a televised session with Senate Democrats, Obama delivered a message of solidarity, assuring the beleaguered lawmakers: "I'm there in the arena with you."

He and the press corps left. Another triumph, it seemed. But then the tensions exploded.

Sen. Al Franken (D-Minn.) launched into a blistering tirade against David Axelrod, a senior White House adviser and one of Obama's closest confidants.

"I have been in a slow burn here, a slow burn," the lawmaker hollered from the last row of the meeting room. "I'm just livid."

Lacing his commentary with profanity, Franken said the health-care campaign had been lackluster and leaderless, particularly in the tentative period since Brown's victory.

"Goddamn it, what's the deal here?" he said, as colleagues, their spouses and aides looked on. "You're talking platitudes, and we have to go home and defend ourselves. We're getting the crap kicked out of us."

Axelrod, a laconic Chicagoan not prone to excitability, catalogued Obama's work over the past year.

"Add up the number of trips, speeches, radio addresses," he said. "I spend a good part of every day with him, and I know that he's still working hard on this issue."

Franken wouldn't relent.

"The president of the United States comes up here, you come here, and none of you are telling us what we're going to do about health care," he continued. "He should apologize to everyone here for his stupid idea during the campaign to put this all on C-SPAN."

To some in the room, Franken's outburst felt like theater from a longtime performer. But others were pleased that the former comedian was giving voice to the months of friction.

"There's a great deal of frustration that the president isn't getting the feelings that a lot of us are feeling," said Sen. Bill Nelson (D-Fla.). "The president needs to be more hands-on with the health-care bill."

"I assure you the president is getting that message," Axelrod replied. "We have a plan."

That set off Sen. Carl M. Levin (D-Mich.).

"What is it? What exactly is the plan?" the onetime lawyer asked in a prosecutorial tone. "What is the strategy?"

Axelrod absorbed the verbal punches—until Franken questioned Obama's commitment to the bill they had spent 12 months selling.

"Al, you can say whatever you want, but don't tell me the president hasn't led on health care," Axelrod said. "This thing would have been dead 15 times before now if he hadn't been persistent and committed. I don't know anybody in my memory who has expended more of his own political capital on an issue than he has on this one."

"Then why doesn't he go over to the House and tell them to pass the Senate bill?" Franken said.

"Al, if you've got 218 votes in your pocket, hand me the list," Axelrod replied. "I will personally walk it over to the speaker and we can take care of this tomorrow. But I don't think she has that list in her pocket."

* * *

By late February, Obama was still on his elusive search for bipartisanship.

In so many ways since taking office, he had seemed to be searching for the right balance between two versions of himself: Obama the idealistic community organizer, and Obama the pragmatic president who could abandon core principles in the drive to pass a bill. He already had reversed course on a requirement that every American carry insurance and given up on a public insurance option.

His decision to hold the bipartisan summit was based in the belief that he could overcome the ferocious partisanship gripping Washington and woo a few Republicans, or at least show that he was trying.

It also brought together the two Obamas.

On Feb. 25, the president and 28 lawmakers squeezed around a giant square of tables in the Garden Room of Blair House. After more than seven hours of talking, the members of Congress grabbed their overcoats and raced for the doors.

Not Obama. He lingered behind, shaking hands, making one last pitch for his stalled initiative. After all the others were gone, he stepped out into the brisk darkness and made the short walk across the street to the White House.

"There were some good things that came out of that," he told advisers in the Oval Office afterward. He said he wanted the final legislation to incorporate a handful of ideas Republicans raised during the session.

A few aides protested. Shouldn't they extract a few votes in return? "Let's bargain for these," one said.

Obama—naively, some would say—still held out hope for a couple of converts. "We're going to accept some of these," he said.

Over the following weekend, DeParle and other administration officials made overtures to several Republicans. They spoke to Rep. Peter Roskam (Ill.), who served with Obama in the state legislature. They conferred with Rep. John Shadegg (Ariz.) about ways to sell insurance across state lines, and Sen. Tom Coburn (Okla.) about his idea to hire "undercover" Medicare fraud investigators.

But it was too late. Republicans denounced the summit as an 11th-hour publicity stunt and declared that they would not help pass Obama's massive health-care bill, even if it did include some of their proposals.

Pelosi, meanwhile, had grown more bullish about her prospects in the House. Though the summit had not won over any Republicans, it had reassured some jittery Democrats that Obama was finally fully engaged in the fight.

The strategy of coming across as a leader appeared to be working. Heartened, Obama now set on what would be the final course of his top domestic priority.

During an appearance in the East Room on March 3, surrounded by doctors in white lab coats, he outlined a final healthcare bill. The substance of his announcement was hardly newsworthy: The Obama proposal was largely a compromise he had helped negotiate in early January, before the election in Massachusetts.

Far more significant was the strategic decision the president made to pursue a delicate procedural two-step that Emanuel and Deputy Chief of Staff Jim Messina had first brought up soon after Brown's Senate victory. Step one: The House would adopt the Senate measure—the very bill that Pelosi had called a "nonstarter." Step two: The House would then approve a batch of changes in a separate budget "reconciliation" bill, which would require only a simple majority of 51 votes in the Senate, not the 60 needed to overcome a filibuster. Even with Brown added to the Republican side, there were still 59 Democrats in the Senate. More than enough.

Democrats, in other words, would go it alone.

* * *

A few hours after his speech in the East Room, Obama threw a party with an ulterior motive.

Under a 19th-century French chandelier, he and a few dozen lawmakers toasted the enactment of a law imposing "pay as you go" budget restrictions. As tuxedoed waiters passed hors d'oeuvres and a bartender poured drinks, Obama, Vice President Biden and a trio of senior advisers worked the room, moving from one clutch of Democratic deficit hawks to another.

The search for votes was on.

In one corner, Biden reminisced about the late congressman John P. Murtha (D-Pa.) with Democratic Reps. Jason Altmire (Pa.), Peter Welch (Vt.) and Lincoln Davis (Tenn.). The president ambled up to the group and praised the lawmakers' support of the legislation, dubbed Paygo.

"This is so extraordinarily important for the country. We have to get back in fiscal balance," Obama said. "Paygo is the tool to help us."

The real reason for the president's schmoozing, however, quickly became evident. Looking at Welch, an enthusiastic supporter of a health-care overhaul, he said: "And you know what else would help us with the deficit?"

Without missing a beat, Welch turned to Altmire, who voted against the bill in November but was on the fence in March, and considered "gettable" by the White House vote-counters.

"Yes," Welch said, "health-care reform."

Then Obama draped one arm over Altmire's shoulder, turned away from the others and leaned in close.

"Peter's right, Jason," he said. "We have to do this. It is essential to bringing down the deficit."

Estimates by the independent Congressional Budget Office would soon show that the measure would reduce the deficit, Obama said, while the status quo "blows the deficit."

Altmire, more than most in Congress, understood the intricacies of health-care policy. As a congressional aide in the 1990s, he had worked on Clinton's failed effort and later became a hospital executive. He opposed the bill in November in part because it would not have gone far enough to control rising medical costs.

Obama saw that as his opening, pointing out to Altmire that the new version would create a Medicare cost-cutting commission.

Altmire reminded Obama that he had been to the congressman's district in western Pennsylvania, a conservative region where Republicans often win and the Roman Catholic bishop holds considerable sway.

"I want to represent my district," he told the president. "As you know, it is politically split."

As Obama drifted toward a lectern to address the entire room, Emanuel made a beeline for Altmire and cornered him. The two went back to Altmire's first congressional race in 2006.

"Your constituents like you; you've built up a reservoir of goodwill," Emanuel said. "You have an opportunity before this vote to go back home and explain it to them."

Obama and Emanuel had made clear that they needed the votes of many of the lawmakers sipping cocktails that evening, even skeptics such as Altmire.

The conversations in the Blue Room, however, were but a gentle hint of what was to come.

* * *

The day after the reception, Obama began his final, most intensive push to corral votes, a round-the-clock effort in which he delved into arcane policy discussions, promised future favors, mapped out election strategy and, when all else failed, painted the grim portrait of what a weakened presidency would mean for Democrats and their lofty legislative ambitions.

He hit the road, rolling up his sleeves at boisterous rallies in suburban Philadelphia, St. Louis and Fairfax, Va. He revived his attacks on the unpopular insurance industry, a strategy bolstered by the latest round of double-digit premium increases. His Cabinet members wrote op-ed pieces, while his political operatives coordinated a $7.6 million pro-reform advertising blitz in 40 targeted congressional districts.

But it was the personal touch—in carefully tailored appeals— that mattered the most in the closing days.

Some fence-sitters nearly drowned in presidential attention. The day after the party in the Blue Room, Altmire was back at the White House for a meeting with centrists in the New Democrat Coalition.

"The economy's going to turn around," Obama assured the

group. With time, he said, "this is going to be viewed as a good vote."

A few lawmakers chimed in to agree, but Rep. Adam Smith (D-Wash.) told Obama that the bill wasn't selling well in some parts of the country. It wasn't simply a matter of "all hold hands and jump off the cliff together," he said, half in jest. "This is going to be difficult."

"If this was easy," the president replied, looking around the Oval Office, "you wouldn't be sitting here."

That same day, Obama faced a group of disillusioned liberals, many of them supporters of a single-payer, government-run health-care system. They had such high hopes that he would stick to his promise to create a public insurance option.

"This is a foundation," he told them. "Thirty-one million Americans will be covered under this. It's a beginning."

Most in the room had already resigned themselves to the Obama compromise, but Rep. Dennis Kucinich (D-Ohio), refused.

"I'm concerned this is going to create a foundation for the increased privatization of the system," he said from a leather chair beneath a "Rough Rider" portrait of Theodore Roosevelt. "It's giving $70 billion to industry."

Kucinich left the White House saddened. He had developed a bond with Obama during the 2008 Democratic presidential primaries and didn't enjoy saying no to his former rival. It appeared they were at an impasse.

The White House had better luck with Rep. Melissa Bean (D-Ill.). After one group meeting, Obama asked her to stay behind.

"Let me talk to my homegirl," he joked. They compared notes on their families—both have two daughters. Then Obama made a gentle plea: "These reforms are really important."

A few days later, seated at the conference table in his spacious corner office, Emanuel was more direct, reminding Bean of the support he lent in her campaigns—and why she came to Washington.

"You ran because you care about the deficit," he said. "This is north of $1 trillion in deficit reduction" over 20 years.

Bean wanted to see the final measure and a cost estimate.

"The Senate bill is stronger than the House bill, and you voted for the House bill," Emanuel volleyed.

"I'm glad you heard us," she replied.

"Melissa, name me once in the last six years you voted for a bill with more deficit reduction," he said. And, he added, if she opposed the legislation, "don't ever send me another press release about deficit reduction."

On Monday, March 15, Obama began what aides hoped would be the final week in their year-long march. On the flight to a rally in Strongsville, Ohio, Kucinich rode with Obama in his private cabin aboard Air Force One.

Seated across a small table with a laptop beside him, Obama ticked off a litany of groundbreaking legislative achievements—all of which, he argued, began small. Medicare, he said. Civil rights.

They hashed through the substance; Obama spoke about the tens of millions of uninsured Americans who would be covered under the bill. It was cordial, but they were still at loggerheads.

Finally, the president recalled that it was Kucinich, in the earliest days of the presidential campaign, who directed his Iowa delegates to back Obama on a second ballot. "Dennis, you were the only candidate to do that," he said.

Now, Obama said, his presidency was on the line. This wasn't about him, "but about our ability to get anything done."

On Capitol Hill, meanwhile, Pelosi was methodically working down her tally sheet, just as she had in early November. This time, because of retirements and Murtha's death, she would need to deliver 216 votes. On Wednesday, she received a pleasant surprise: Kucinich had changed his position.

The Ohioan's support was more than just one vote in the "yes" column; it was the start of the momentum the White House had been struggling to create.

In short order, the good news rolled out in a steady, well-choreographed clip.

"Gordon, Markey, join 'no' to 'yes'" contingent, one announcement said. "Boccieri switches to 'yes,' " said another, referring to Rep. John Boccieri (D-Ohio). At the White House, confident aides stole time to watch the NCAA basketball tournament.

Obama, meanwhile, doused a brush fire with organized labor over changes to a new excise tax that unions did not like. After a chance encounter in Messina's office that was actually well planned out, Obama pulled AFL-CIO President Richard Trumka into the Oval Office.

"We're at the one-yard line. We've just got to get the ball in the end zone," the president said, imploring Trumka to hold his complaints for another day. "Rich, you've got to stay with me."

But not everything went their way, and Pelosi and Obama sweated into the weekend.

On Friday morning, Altmire e-mailed Emanuel. Despite a second party at the White House on St. Patrick's Day, a sit-down with Emanuel, a few more phone calls from the president and three from Cabinet-level officials, Altmire planned to announce that he would vote no.

"Don't do it," Emanuel punched back on his BlackBerry. At 4 p.m., Altmire released his statement and at 7:30 Obama called once more.

"I want to give you something to think about before the vote," the president said gently into the phone. "Picture yourself on Monday morning. You wake up and look at the paper. It's the greatest thing Congress has done in 50 years. And you were on the wrong team." But the lawmaker wasn't going to change his mind.

Saturday now. Two days left, and it was time for the closing strategy. Arm twist after arm twist, deal after deal, the final days played out so publicly that at some point amid the news conferences and speeches it started to feel like a compressed, frenetic rehashing of the entire fight.

Protesters on the Capitol lawn. Rumors of enticements—a Cabinet post, water access in California, money for NASA. More phone calls, more news conferences, frayed nerves, exhaustion.

At the Capitol, Pelosi was once again dealing with the specter of abortion funding, shuttling from office to office as she locked down the votes once again.

And Obama, once again, was ensconced in the White House contemplating the fate of his signature domestic initiative, a scene so familiar that it could have been Jan. 19 all over again.

But this time, instead of panic, instead of sniping and interrupting, there was a victory.

Obama had done it, and toward midnight on March 21, 2010, he said to the American people:

"In the end, what this day represents is another stone firmly laid in the foundation of the American dream. Tonight, we answered the call of history as so many generations of Americans have before us. When faced with crisis, we did not shrink from our challenge—we overcame it. We did not avoid our responsibility—we embraced it. We did not fear our future—we shaped it."

Here came health-care reform.

Here came history.

PART II

WHAT IT MEANS FOR US ALL

By
Alec MacGillis
David Brown
Howard Gleckman
Amy Goldstein
David S. Hilzenrath
Lori Montgomery
Shailagh Murray

Rising Spending

Controlling costs is one of the goals of overhauling the U.S. health-care system.

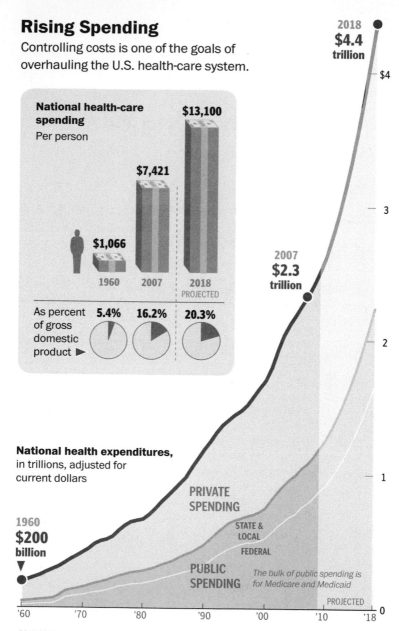

National health-care spending
Per person

$1,066 — 1960
$7,421 — 2007
$13,100 — 2018 PROJECTED

As percent of gross domestic product ▶
5.4% — 16.2% — 20.3%

National health expenditures, in trillions, adjusted for current dollars

2018 $4.4 trillion

2007 $2.3 trillion

1960 $200 billion

PRIVATE SPENDING

STATE & LOCAL

FEDERAL

PUBLIC SPENDING

The bulk of public spending is for Medicare and Medicaid

PROJECTED

'60 '70 '80 '90 '00 '10 '18

SOURCE: Department of Health and Human Services

The Best, the Worst, the Future

Start with this contradiction.

American medicine remains the envy of the world. The United States has many of the best hospitals. It has well-trained, highly skilled and innovative doctors. It produces the lion's share of the most significant advances in biomedical research.

Yet the same country has constructed a health-care system that is wasteful, inefficient, increasingly irrational—and unsustainably expensive. We spend a fortune on medical care, and yet we're lagging behind other nations in several major categories that define a healthy country.

We devote about 17 percent of our gross domestic product to health care, far more than any other developed nation. Despite such high spending, millions of us do not receive the care we need. Unlike every other wealthy industrialized democracy, ours does not guarantee health insurance. According to the U.S. Census Bureau, more than 45 million of us lack coverage.

No one seems immune from the system's ailments. The 59 percent of us with employer-provided insurance have watched our coverage diminish even as our costs continue to rise. The 18 million or so of us who buy coverage on the private market often find ourselves in a running battle with insurers over medical claims—assuming we even find affordable plans, which is unlikely for those with a preexisting condition. Small businesses struggle to provide health coverage for their workers, lacking the ability to spread insurance risk as broadly as large employers can. Medical bills are a leading factor in more than half the country's personal bankruptcies, studies show. The United States ranks 31st in the world for life expectancy and 37th for infant mortality, according to the World Health Organization.

Meanwhile, the surge in spending shows no sign of abating. The Congressional Budget Office predicted recently that absent major changes, health-care costs would swell to 25 percent of the economy in 2025, 37 percent in 2050 and 49 percent in 2082. There are sociological and demographic explanations for this breathtaking ratio: As societies grow wealthier, it is only natural that people spend more of their money on trying to stay healthy and live longer. Evidence suggests that when it comes to end-of-life care, we Americans are even more insistent than our peers in Europe and Asia in trying to ward off mortality. In addition, the country struggles with high levels of costly conditions such as obesity and diabetes.

Whatever the driver of our health-care spending, though, it is threatening to ruin our finances and swallow our economy. The country's fiscal woes—the CBO projects the federal public debt will reach $20 trillion, 90 percent of gross domestic product, by 2020— are rooted above all in the burgeoning costs of Medicare and Medicaid, with the baby-boomer retirement wave still looming. The rising cost of insurance contributes to the stagnation of our wages. Every dollar that goes into health care means less to invest in engines of growth such as education, infrastructure and renewable energy.

Welcome to the (Complicated) Future

This is the flawed system that the Patient Protection and Affordable Care Act of 2010 seeks to overhaul. The legislation will cost nearly $1 trillion over its first 10 years, which it seeks to pay for through taxes, industry fees and spending cuts. It is the biggest expansion of the social safety net in more than four decades, providing greater economic security to millions of poor and working-class

Falling Behind

The United States spends far more per person than other industrialized nations, but that doesn't necessarily result in better care.

2006 data

Per-capita health expenditures

Japan	$2,578
Britain	2,760
Germany	3,371
Canada	3,678
United States	6,714

Preventable deaths per 100,000 population

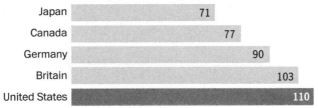

Japan	71
Canada	77
Germany	90
Britain	103
United States	110

Infant deaths per 1,000 live births

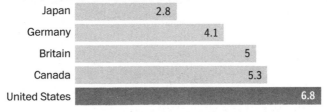

Japan	2.8
Germany	4.1
Britain	5
Canada	5.3
United States	6.8

SOURCE: Alliance for Health Reform, Organization for Economic Co-operation and Development, Commonwealth Fund

families. It will reach into almost every corner of the health-care system.

But for all its scope, the law is a relatively moderate and incremental document—evolutionary, not revolutionary. It does not seek to replace the country's system of private health insurance with a government-run, "single-payer" system such as Canada's—the "Medicare for all" approach advocated by many American liberals for years, but sharply opposed by insurers and many medical providers. It will not dismantle or fundamentally alter the system of employer-based insurance, as several alternative proposals would have done by tossing aside the tax-free treatment of employer benefits. And it does not go nearly so far as President Bill Clinton's failed plan in 1993–94 in trying to set insurance premium levels and medical provider rates.

Instead, the law seeks to expand the number of people covered and begin the work of restraining costs by building on the existing structure of private insurance. This market-based approach bears clear resemblance to the leading Republican alternative to the Clinton plan, to proposals developed by the conservative Heritage Foundation, and to the 2006 legislation signed by Republican Mitt Romney that created universal coverage in Massachusetts.

Like the Massachusetts approach, the new federal law seeks to achieve near-universal coverage with a three-part formula. It requires insurers to provide coverage to anyone who wants it. To make it feasible for insurers to offer coverage to people with existing medical conditions, it requires everyone to obtain health insurance, thereby broadening the risk pool to include both the healthy and less healthy. And, to make sure that people can afford the insurance they will be required to have, it provides subsidies to help them buy private insurance.

The centerpiece of all this will be new "exchanges," state-based marketplaces where, starting in 2014, small businesses and people without employer-based insurance will be able to shop for plans that meet the law's standards. Insurers will have access to millions of new customers, as long as they follow the new rules. The exchanges will not include the much-debated "public option"—or government-run plan—that, as its proponents saw it, would have competed with private insurers and brought considerable bargaining power to bear in seeking lower rates from medical providers.

Despite its relatively straightforward approach to expanding coverage, the law is dense and complex, much like the sprawling, interlocking, convoluted system that it seeks to reshape. Part Two of *Landmark* takes a comprehensive look at the new law, not just what it means for individual consumers and their medical care, but what it means for the health-care system and its component parts: doctors, hospitals, Medicare, Medicaid, large employers and small employers, states and insurers.

It's a guide to what Congress did, and didn't, accomplish. It addresses many of the major questions in detail. Among them: How will people without employer-based coverage obtain insurance? What does the law mean for people who already have coverage? How is the law paid for? What does it require of employers? What effect will it have on the way doctors and hospitals do their work?

It also draws attention to some of the unresolved issues that will hang over the law as it is implemented. For all the time that went into drafting the law, much remains unknown: Will people comply with a mandate to obtain insurance? Will Congress follow through on the cuts and taxes the law calls for? Will the attempts to change the way we deliver care rein in the seemingly relentless rise in spending on our health? What are the key areas of contention as federal regulators begin the task of writing the all-important rules that will spell out how to implement the legislation?

The new law, for good or ill, in ways big and small, will affect us all. What follows is a guide to help you navigate the evolving, uncertain (but certainly complicated) landscape that lies ahead.

— Alec MacGillis

Implementation Timeline

When some of the major provisions of the health-care law will kick in:

2010-2013: INTERIM MEASURES

	2010	2011	2012
TAXES/FEES	Tax credit available for some small businesses to help provide coverage for workers. Indoor tanning services taxed 10 percent.	Employers required to disclose value of health benefits on W-2 tax forms. Annual fee imposed on pharmaceutical companies. Chain restaurants and food sold from vending machines must disclose nutritional content.	
EXPANSION OF COVERAGE	Uninsured adults with preexisting conditions can get health coverage as part of a "high risk pool." Insurance companies are banned from denying coverage to children with pre-existing conditions, dropping coverage when someone gets sick and placing lifetime limits on coverage. Adult children up to age 26 can stay on their parent's coverage plan. Temporary reinsurance program helps companies maintain coverage for early retirees between the ages of 55 and 64.	For drugs bought in the Medicare Part D coverage gap: Drug manufacturers will be required to provide a 50% discount on brand-name; generic benefit will start at an extra 7% this year, rising to 75% by 2020. Medicare will start 10% bonus payments to primary care physicians and general surgeons. Payments to private health plans offering Medicare Advantage services are frozen at 2010 levels.	Payment rates start to be reduced for Medicare Advantage plans. The Centers for Medicare and Medicaid Services begins tracking hospital readmission rates and puts in place financial incentives to reduce preventable readmissions.
MEDICARE/ MEDICAID	Medicare drug beneficiaries who fall into the "doughnut hole" coverage gap get a $250 rebate.	States can offer home- and community- based care for the disabled under Medicaid.	

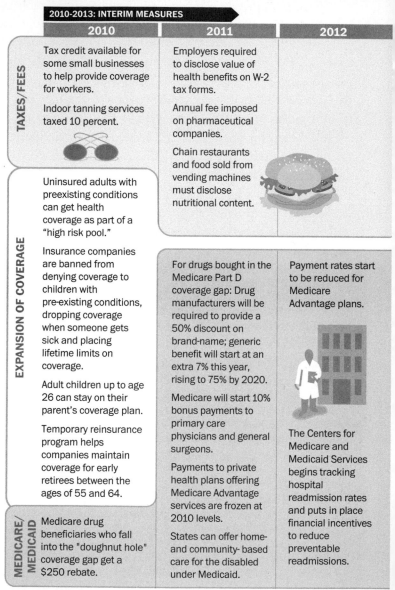

SOURCE: Kaiser Family Foundation

EXCHANGES AND OTHER MAJOR INITIATIVES BEGIN

2013	2014	2015-2018	
Threshold for claiming medical expenses on itemized tax returns is raised to 10% from 7.5% of income. Contributions to flexible spending accounts limited to $2,500 per year. A 2.9% excise tax is imposed on sale of medical devices.	Employers with 50 or more workers who do not offer coverage face a fine of $2,000 for each employee if any worker receives subsidized insurance in the exchange. The first 30 employees aren't counted for the fine. Insurance companies begin paying a fee based on their market share.	**2018** An excise tax is imposed on employer-provided plans that cost more than $10,200 for an individual or $27,500 for a family.	**TAXES/FEES**
Medicare payroll tax raised to 2.35% for individuals earning more than $200,000 and married couples with incomes over $250,000. A 3.8% tax is imposed on investment income. Federal subsidies begin for brand-name prescriptions bought in the Medicare Part D coverage gap.	State-based insurance exchanges open for business. Premium credits and cost-sharing subsidies become available to help people with incomes up to 400 percent of the federal poverty level buy coverage in the exchange. Health plans are banned from excluding people with preexisting conditions. Most people are required to obtain insurance or pay a fine.		**EXPANSION OF COVERAGE**
	Medicaid expands to all individuals younger than 65 with incomes up to 133 percent of the federal poverty level.	**2015** Medicare creates a physician payment program aimed at rewarding quality of care rather than volume of services.	**MEDICARE/ MEDICAID**

CHAPTER 1

Priority One: Expanding Coverage

Helping Americans get affordable, adequate health insurance stands as the central goal of the Patient Protection and Affordable Care Act. The law will, if Congress's budget analysts turn out to be right, lead to coverage for 32 million more people in the United States, starting in 2014.

The law does not quite strive for universal coverage, the Holy Grail for proponents of the most ambitious health-care reform. Still, it tries to make the biggest dent in the country's uninsured population that the government has ever attempted in a single step. If it works, 95 percent of U.S. citizens and other legal residents will have insurance within six years. The law's strategies are aimed mainly at people who cannot obtain or afford coverage through a workplace, because their employer does not offer any or because it is too expensive—or because they are unemployed or work for themselves.

The new law settles, at least for now, a decades-old debate over whether the government should be in the business of providing insurance directly or of helping people buy private policies. The verdict? The law does some of each.

- It opens the doors of Medicaid, the government health insurance program for the poor, to people who could not join before.
- It creates insurance "exchanges," the government's name for newfangled marketplaces aimed at people who cannot obtain affordable coverage through a job or on their own. If the idea works as intended, the exchanges will help people get better coverage at lower prices and make it easier to shop for it.
- It provides federal subsidies to most people who buy insurance through an exchange.

Here's how each part is supposed to work:

Opening Medicaid's Doors

Almost half of the estimated 32 million Americans expected to gain insurance will do so through Medicaid, created in 1965, when President Lyndon B. Johnson was in the White House. Starting in 2014, the federal government will, for the first time, specify who can join Medicaid, rather than leaving it largely up to each state. The government will also guarantee that a package of "essential health services" be available for Medicaid recipients, no matter where they live, though states will be able to offer more, if they choose.

Two big new groups of people will be helped.

Adults without dependent children. In most states, they have been shut out of Medicaid until now.

People with incomes a bit higher than most states have allowed in the past. Every U.S. citizen and legal resident younger than age 65 will qualify for Medicaid if they have an income of up to 133 percent of the federal poverty line—in 2010, $14,404 for a single adult or $29,327 for a family of four.

The federal government will play a much bigger role in paying

WHAT'S THE BIG PROBLEM?

The uninsured population in the United States has been increasing almost every year, rising from about 38 million to 46 million in the past decade alone. More people now lack health-care coverage, in large part because it has become more expensive. The result? Fewer employers have been offering it. Even when they do, an increasing number of people, particularly young adults who tend to be healthy, have decided it is not worth the cost. Plus, in the recent bad economy, people have been losing jobs—and their health coverage, too.

Although specific forecasts vary, many experts say that, if the government had not stepped in, the number of people without coverage would have kept growing. Recent research by the Urban Institute, a Washington think tank, suggests that the total number of uninsured adults younger than 65 would have reached 58 million to 68 million within the next decade, with the increase concentrated among the middle class.

Having health insurance does not, on its own, guarantee good care. It does not, for example, ensure that people will have nearby access to doctors with the needed skills. But many studies over the years have shown that uninsured people are less likely to receive the treatment they need, especially if they have a serious or chronic medical problem.

for Medicaid, a financial responsibility it has always shared with the states. The federal government also will pay the states more to run an existing program, the Children's Health Insurance Program. The eligibility rules for CHIP, set largely by the states, will not change.

Shopping at an Exchange

The new exchanges—one of the most significant ways in which the law will change the health-care system—will start in 2014. By

2018, about 24 million people will be buying their insurance this way, according to government predictions. The basic concept is to make it easier for those eligible for the exchanges to find affordable plans and to comparison-shop.

The exchanges are supposed to do this in two ways:

- Reducing rates by "pooling" the medical risks of people who otherwise would be looking for insurance on their own or as part of a small group of workers—two sets of consumers for whom coverage has been particularly expensive until now.
- Requiring insurance companies to offer certain standard benefits and levels of coverage, so that people have an easier time comparing plans and prices.

To accomplish all this, states must, by the beginning of 2014, create an American Health Benefit Exchange. Most states will have one exchange, but exceptions are likely. The law allows larger states to have more than one, while sparsely populated states could band together with neighbors to create regional exchanges.

States also must create a small-business exchange for companies with 100 employees or fewer. Starting in 2017, the states may, if they choose, allow larger employers to purchase coverage through a small-business exchange. States can merge their small-business exchange with the other exchange if they want to.

The exchanges must be run by a state agency or a nonprofit organization. They will be doing a lot of complicated work behind the scenes with the insurance industry and two federal agencies, but most of that is supposed to be invisible to consumers.

To shop for coverage, people can visit an exchange office near them, go to the exchange's Web site or call a toll-free helpline. The exchange will determine whether the consumers qualify to buy insurance this way and whether they are eligible for a federal subsidy. (For more about the subsidies, see the next section, Getting a Subsidy.)

MORE BUREAUCRACY?

A House aide who helped write the parts of the law dealing with the new exchanges said the authors put a big priority on making it easy for consumers to sign up and to find out whether they qualify for government subsidies.

The exchanges are not as much "big government" as a single-payer health-care system would have been, or even as one nationwide exchange, which Congress considered and rejected.

But here's one clue to the scale of the task ahead: Congressional budget analysts predict that it will cost the Internal Revenue Service $5 billion to $10 billion in the first decade to determine which Americans are eligible for the new subsidies.

The law does not say how many plans must be offered through each exchange, but the idea is that there should be choices—a variety of insurance companies and a variety of coverage levels offered by the same insurer. For the most part, health plans will differ from state to state. But the federal government will choose two private plans that must be sold nationwide.

To help people compare plans, a new standardized system will spell out the coverage levels that insurers offer. This system will have four tiers: "bronze" at the low end, then "silver," "gold" and—at the high end, with the most coverage—"platinum." (See chart on following page for an explanation of the tiers.) Each tier refers to a specific percentage of a person's medical costs that a plan must, on average, cover. In addition to the tiers, the government is creating a quality-rating system that also is intended to help with comparison-shopping.

Exchanges will not set insurance rates. But if a state's regulators conclude that an insurer has raised prices too high, they will have the power to bar that insurer from the exchange.

The Four Tiers of Coverage

To standardize coverage and make comparison-shopping easier, the law specifies new tiers of coverage that will be available through the exchanges. The law creates four possible tiers, plus a low-cost, bare-bones "catastrophic" plan for those who are younger than 30 and those who are exempt from the requirement to buy an insurance plan. Insurers must offer silver and gold tiers to participate in the exchanges; they have the option to include bronze and platinum plans as well.

Plans MUST offer silver and gold tier coverage

Bronze plan	Silver plan	Gold plan	Platinum plan
 60% covered	 70% covered	 80% covered	90% covered
Provides the essential health benefits as defined by the government. It covers **60%** of the cost of the plan's benefits, with an out-of-pocket limit equal to the Health Savings Account (HSA) current limit ($5,950 for individuals and $11,900 for families in 2010).	Provides the essential health benefits, and covers **70%** of the cost of the plan's benefits, with the HSA out-of-pocket limits.	Provides the essential health benefits, and covers **80%** of the cost of the plan's benefits, with the HSA out-of-pocket limits.	Provides the essential health benefits, and covers **90%** of the cost of the plan's benefits, with the HSA out-of-pocket limits.

Getting a Subsidy

In 2014, the year the exchanges begin, the federal government will offer unprecedented financial assistance to help people pay for private coverage if they do not qualify for a public insurance program. About 19 million of the 24 million people who use an exchange will receive at least some help, Congress's budget analysts predict. It will come in two forms, and most people who qualify for one will also qualify for the other:

- "Premium credits" to help pay their insurance premiums.
- Subsidies to limit their out-of-pocket spending on deductibles and co-pays.

The amount of financial help will depend on income. People at lower income levels, who just miss the eligibility cut-off for Medicaid, will receive significantly more assistance than those at the higher end, which reaches into the upper middle class.

Here's how the subsidies will work:

Premium credits. People at different income levels will, according to a formula, receive a credit that will reduce the amount they have to pay toward their premium. The government will pay the insurer the difference. The amounts are linked to the price of a "silver" insurance policy, the second-lowest tier of coverage.

The subsidy to limit out-of-pocket spending. Almost all insurance plans require deductibles, co-pays and other forms of cost-sharing. Federal rules will limit the share that consumers in the exchanges must pay. The government will pick up the rest. Again, the subsidy depends on the consumer's income. For the group with the lowest income, for example, the government must cover 94 percent of expenses, leaving the consumer to pay no more than 6 percent.

Subsidizing the Cost of Insurance

The government will provide premium credits and subsidies for out-of-pocket costs to help most of the individuals and families that will buy health insurance on the exchanges. The subsidy size will depend on income. The new law spells out how the subsidies will work:

Scenario 1: Single person

	Premium credits		Subsidies for out-of-pocket costs
INCOME	PREMIUM AS % OF INCOME		% OF OUT-OF-POCKET PAID BY GOVERNMENT

0

If you make between	$14,404	2%*		Covered by Medicaid
	$16,245	3-4%	Your premium would not exceed this percentage of your income	94%
	$21,660	4-6.3%		85%
	$27,075	6.3-8.05%		73%
	$32,490	8.05-9.5%		70%
	$43,320	9.5%		70%
Above		No limit		0

The government would pay this percentage of your out-of-pocket costs

Scenario 2: Family of four

	Premium credits		Subsidies for out-of-pocket costs
INCOME	PREMIUM AS % OF INCOME		% OF OUT-OF-POCKET PAID BY GOVERNMENT

0

If you make between	$29,327	2%*		Covered by Medicaid
	$33,075	3-4%	Your premium would not exceed this percentage of your income	94%
	$44,100	4-6.3%		85%
	$55,125	6.3-8.05%		73%
	$66,150	8.05-9.5%		70%
	$88,200	9.5%		70%
Above		No limit		0

The government would pay this percentage of your out-of-pocket costs

NOTE: The law derives the income level from a percentage above the poverty level
*Legal immigrants barred from enrolling in Medicaid during their first five years in the U.S. will be eligible for premium credits

Who qualifies for subsidies?

Like the exchanges, the subsidies are designed mainly for people who are unable to obtain coverage through a job. But both will be available to people whose employers offer only insurance that is too expensive or doesn't provide enough coverage.

Here's the nitty-gritty: People who have access to employer-based coverage can use the exchanges and receive a subsidy if they meet the regular income requirements and:

1) They would have to pay more than 9.5 percent of their income toward the plan their employer offers, or
2) Their employer's plan covers less than 60 percent, on average, of the benefits it includes.

To apply for a subsidy, consumers will contact the exchange near them and provide income information. If the exchange determines that a person is eligible, it will collect only that part of the premium that the consumer owes. The exchange then files a request with a branch of the Treasury Department, asking it to pay the balance to the insurance company. For the subsidies that help with out-of-pocket costs, the Department of Health and Human Services will send money directly to the insurer.

People will not have to pay up front any part of their insurance that the government will subsidize. There is an exception, though. If someone's income goes down during the course of a year, the government will refund whatever portion the consumer did not really owe. On the other hand, if someone's income goes up, he or she will have to pay the exchange the difference. The exchange will keep tabs on all this.

Swimming in a High-Risk Pool

Because most of the help will not start until 2014, the government is taking a temporary step right away to try to make coverage more affordable for one group that finds it particularly expensive: people who have existing medical problems and have been uninsured for at least six months.

This help will come in the form of a nationwide "high-risk pool," an idea pioneered at the state level. Like the exchanges, the idea is to lower insurance prices by spreading the medical risk for people who find individual coverage too expensive.

The high-risk pool is supposed to begin by June 2010. The Department of Health and Human Services must quickly set the rates and draft various rules, which are meant to be in harmony with the high-risk pools that about three dozen states have created in recent years. Overall, these programs, in which states invest about $2 billion nationwide, have not proved popular. Only about 200,000 people have signed up for them. The reason? They tend to be expensive, and the coverage can be skimpy. To help solve those problems, the government is chipping in $5 billion.

The federal high-risk pool must cover at least 65 percent of participants' care, while limiting out-of-pocket costs to $5,950 a year for an individual or $11,900 for a family in 2010. It remains unclear whether the federal money and the coverage rules will be enough to motivate people to sign up.

Those Left Out

For the first time, most people in the United States will be required to have health insurance, or be fined. But there are exceptions. The requirement does not apply to immigrants living in the U.S. illegally, people in prison, those with certain religious objections, or those uninsured for brief periods. Nor does it apply to Native Americans or military veterans, who receive treatment through their own health-care systems. (See Chapter 2, The Individual Mandate.)

The government predicts that about 23 million people will not have insurance by the end of the decade. Some will not be affected by the individual mandate. Others will somehow not know about the requirement. Still others will refuse to comply, and risk the fine instead.

How Well Will All This Work?

There are many lingering questions about how this approach to expanding insurance coverage will work in practice. Here are two big ones:

- How many people will refuse to get insurance? Experts disagree about whether the fines are big enough—and the government will be tough enough—to bring resisters into the system.
- Will the subsidies provide enough help? The government has never before offered this much aid for buying private insurance. Some experts wonder whether the subsidies are large enough to motivate healthy people to sign up, and enough to keep pace with rising medical costs and insurance prices.

—*Amy Goldstein*

CHAPTER 2

The Individual Mandate: How It Will Work

A simple rule lies at the heart of the Patient Protection and Affordable Care Act: Starting in 2014, almost every American will need to carry health insurance or pay a fine. That rule is known as the individual mandate.

What It Means for You

The mandate requires all citizens and legal immigrants to have "qualifying" health coverage. People eligible for employer coverage can satisfy the requirement by enrolling in their employer's plan. Employer plans will need to meet certain standards—covering preventive care and disallowing lifetime limits—but will not need to have all of the minimum benefits that will be required of plans sold to individuals and small businesses.

People without insurance through their employer will be able to buy plans on new state-based insurance marketplaces called exchanges, where most will qualify for subsidies. The lowest-price conventional insurance plan for sale on the exchanges must meet the minimum standard for qualifying health coverage: It must cover 60 percent of costs, and out-of-pocket expenses must be limited to $5,950 for individuals and $11,900 for families.

Ways People Would Be Insured

Projections, in millions

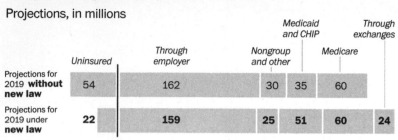

SOURCE: Congressional Budget Office

There is an important exception: People younger than 30 will be able to satisfy the mandate by buying low-cost, high-deductible plans. The plans will require about $6,000 in out-of-pocket spending before most benefits kick in, though they will cover certain screening tests and immunizations before the deductible, and may cover some primary-care visits as well. One advocacy group estimates that premiums for these plans will be $138 per month, compared with $190 per month for the least expensive conventional plan on the exchange. The thinking behind this option is that it will appeal to so-called young invincibles who believe they can do without broader coverage. Insurers argue, though, that if too many young people sign on to these plans, the risk pool in the conventional plans will be weighted too heavily toward older people.

What will happen if I choose not to obtain coverage?

You will be assessed a tax penalty that is the greater of a flat sum or a percent of income: $95 or 1 percent of income in 2014, $325 or 2 percent of income in 2015, and then the penalty's full level in 2016, $695 or 2.5 percent of income. After 2016, the flat dollar amount increases by a cost-of-living adjustment.

For children, the per-person sum is half the adult one. The maximum family penalty is the greater of 2.5 percent of income or three times the per-adult penalty ($2,085 in 2016). All penalties

WHY A MANDATE MATTERS

The thinking behind the individual mandate is that, in the absence of a government-run "single payer" insurance program like Canada's, the only way to achieve universal health insurance is to require people to obtain coverage on their own, with government assistance for those who can't afford it.

Insurance—whether for cars, homes or health—works by spreading the risk. For the tens of millions of Americans who receive health coverage through large employers, the costs are shared broadly: Older workers pay the same as younger workers, and the costs of care are spread across the pool.

But in today's individual insurance market where people without employer-provided coverage buy plans, the spreading of risk does not function so well. About one-third of people age 20 to 29 go without coverage, double the rate for those age 30 to 64. This leaves the individual insurance market dominated by older, sicker people who tend to use more medical care. As a result, rates in the individual market are high, and that, in a kind of vicious cycle, makes it even less likely that younger or healthier people will decide to buy coverage.

Meanwhile, when those without insurance need care, many of the costs end up being borne indirectly by those who are insured: Hospitals and doctors frequently make up the losses by charging other patients more and by relying on government money to help pay for uncompensated care. And because people without insurance often wait longer to seek treatment, the cost of tending to them is higher than it would have been if they had gone in earlier.

This is where the mandate comes in: One of the primary goals of health-care reform is to keep insurance companies from refusing to cover people with preexisting conditions, or from covering them only at exorbitantly high rates. But insurers argue, with justification, that if they have to offer affordable coverage to people with serious medical conditions, then they need to have younger and healthier people in the pool. And the only way to make sure that those people obtain coverage is to require it.

are capped at the cost of the lowest-priced conventional plan on the exchanges.

What if I can't afford coverage?

Hardship exemptions will be granted for those who are truly unable to afford insurance even with the subsidies that will be available—those for whom the least expensive plan option in their area exceeds 8 percent of their income. (See Chapter 1 for more on the subsidies.) People who qualify for the hardship exemption also will be allowed to buy the high-deductible plan through the exchanges, even if they are older than 30.

Are there any exemptions?

People who lack coverage for a short period—up to three months—will not have to pay a penalty.

Exemptions also will be granted to people who choose not to seek medical care because of their religion, to Native Americans who are covered by the Indian Health Program, to veterans who are covered through the Department of Veterans Affairs, and to people in jail or prison.

Illegal immigrants will not be subject to the mandate, nor will they be allowed to buy insurance through the exchanges. They will instead have to purchase coverage from companies that are still selling plans outside the exchanges, where government regulations and consumer protections will be lighter. They will be able to seek care, as they do now, at federally funded community health clinics and in hospital emergency rooms.

Hospitals that treat large numbers of poor patients will receive less federal support than they do now, on the rationale that more of their patients will be covered. But they will still get some aid in recognition of the fact that many immigrants will remain uncovered, and that some of their other patients will, at least at the outset, not obtain coverage. Whether that aid proves adequate remains to be seen—particularly in states such as California and Texas, where as many as 25 percent of residents are uninsured and there are high numbers of illegal immigrants.

What will happen if I do not obtain coverage or pay the fine?

Some opponents of the legislation conjured images of the government rounding up people and sending them to jail. But the law expressly states that failure to pay the penalties will not result in criminal prosecution or even in property liens. Also, the government probably will enforce the mandate loosely because of the political sensitivity of the health-care law. In fact, those who wrote the legislation set the penalty for not carrying health coverage lower than what many health-care experts believe is necessary for the mandate to work, precisely because they were worried about the political fallout from making the requirement seem too onerous.

Will It Work?

The relatively small penalty and the prospect of loose enforcement create a big potential problem: If many younger and healthier people decide to pay the fine instead of buying coverage, rates will increase for those who do buy it.

Some health-care experts argue that the government will need to adopt a different approach. One option: Encourage everyone to obtain insurance but present those who do not with a choice. They could pay a much larger penalty than the one in the new law, while still retaining the ability to seek subsidized coverage if they do become sick; or they could sign a form on their tax return acknowledging that they were not insured and would therefore be ineligible for a fixed period—say, five years—for federal subsidies or for the protections in the law that allow people to buy coverage even if they have preexisting conditions. This would leave them facing a market with all the uncertainties of the current one. But creating an opt-out of this sort would address critics' concerns about the propriety or political risk of requiring people to have insurance.

The Massachusetts experiment

Some of the law's supporters take heart in Massachusetts's experience with the individual mandate. Since that state adopted universal coverage in 2006, it has managed to get all but about 3 percent of its population insured. But Massachusetts started with a much higher percentage of the population covered than the rest of the country—9 percent of its residents were uninsured in 2006, compared with 15 percent in the entire United States now.

How did Massachusetts get to 97 percent coverage? The state government—working with hospitals, insurers and community groups—began an aggressive campaign to inform the public about the mandate and encourage compliance. The goal was to get people to think of having health insurance as a social norm, not unlike wearing a seatbelt—something they would do because it was right and expected, regardless of the penalty for noncompliance.

The state made it easy to sign up: People who qualified for subsidized coverage received help filling out forms at hospitals and clinics, while others could use a Web site to determine whether they qualified for subsidies or could telephone the Health Connector, the state's version of the exchanges in the new federal law.

Residents were deluged with publicity. The Boston Red Sox promoted the mandate, pharmacy loudspeakers intoned it, grocery store receipts carried reminders and churches coaxed congregants. The Health Connector held 200 meetings with employers and two dozen outreach sessions; community groups received funding to help people sign up; and residents received red-lettered postcards in the mail.

It worked. A Health Connector board member said that a typical comment from young adults coming to apply for coverage was: "My mom said I had to sign up for health insurance or I would get into trouble."

But Jon Kingsdale, the program's executive director, says he worries about the prospects for duplicating the state's success nationally. He thinks the penalty in the federal law is insufficient—in Massachusetts, the fine started at $219 and rose above $1,000 in 2010.

In addition, Massachusetts residents are accustomed to an activist state government, and the mandate was part of a law that had bipartisan support. It was signed by a Republican governor, Mitt Romney, who wrote in 2006: "Some of my libertarian friends balk at what looks like an individual mandate. But remember, someone has to pay for the health care that must, by law, be provided: Either the individual pays or the taxpayers pay. A free ride on the government is not libertarian."

Political challenges

The national mandate will be implemented in a far more toxic political environment, making it more difficult for the government to create a nationwide expectation of compliance. The administration plans to start a promotional campaign as 2014 nears, much as George W. Bush's administration promoted the new Medicare drug benefit.

Within weeks of the signing several legal challenges were already in the works from state attorneys general arguing that it is unconstitutional to require people to buy a given product, in this case health insurance. Most constitutional law experts, including those with conservative leanings, say that the mandate is constitutional, falling under the powers granted the federal government to impose taxes and to regulate interstate commerce.

Whatever the lawsuits' outcome, the momentum behind them

suggests that come 2014, regardless of whether Democrats hold on to the White House, there will be deep pockets of resistance to the mandate. This could seriously complicate the implementation of a health-care program that relies so much on the premise that everyone obtain coverage.

— *Alec MacGillis*

CHAPTER 3

The Insurers: More Customers, More Restrictions

The new law not only provides billions of dollars per year in subsidies to help millions more Americans afford coverage, it also revamps the rules that govern insurers, and in particular the policies they sell to people who do not receive coverage through their employers.

Changes in Fall 2010

In September 2010, six months after the law's enactment, the insurance industry will be subject to three major new rules:

1) Insurers will face sharp restrictions on rescission. This is the highly controversial practice of revoking coverage after a person files a claim. Typically, it involves finding a misstatement on the original insurance application and citing it as a reason to revoke the policy, even if the misstatement is minor or has no bearing on the new illness. As of September, insurers can rescind coverage only in cases of outright fraud by the enrollee.
2) Insurers will no longer be able to deny coverage to children with preexisting conditions. Immediately after the bill was signed into law, uncertainty arose over what this provision actually meant: The legislation's language made it sound as

93

though insurers would no longer be able to deny covering children for treatment of conditions that predated the issuance of the insurance policy, but that they might still be permitted to refuse to sell policies to families because of a child's preexisting condition. The Health and Human Services Department has now said that it will make clear that both practices will be banned.

3) Insurers will no longer be able to impose lifetime limits on benefits paid out. This rule affects people buying plans on the individual insurance market and those with coverage through their jobs, because an increasing number of employer-provided plans now include lifetime limits.

Limits on Insurance-Rate Increases

What will keep insurers from raising rates for individual policies very sharply before the new insurance exchanges debut in 2014? That is a definite concern, but the law includes a provision intended to reduce the chances of this happening: Starting in 2011, insurers will need to spend a minimum percentage of their income from premiums on medical care, instead of keeping that money as profit or to pay for administrative overhead. As it now stands, these "medical loss ratios" are sometimes as low as 70 percent, and in many states, insurers are not required to disclose them. Starting in January 2011, insurers on the individual market will need to spend at least 80 percent of premiums on medical care, and those on the employer-based market will need to spend at least 85 percent. Those with lower medical-loss ratios will have to send their customers rebates to make up the difference.

How effective this rule will be at preventing big rate increases will depend on how federal officials write the new regulations. Insurers have become adept at classifying some overhead costs as medical spending, thereby making their ratios look higher. The law also contains language that gives regulators authority to bar

BRINGING ORDER TO THE WILD WEST

As it now stands, Americans who try to buy insurance for themselves confront a Wild West of high prices and lax or inscrutable consumer protection.

In heavily regulated states in the Northeast, it can be hard to find inexpensive plans, because insurers are required to pay for a wide array of procedures and are constrained in their ability to vary rates based on the consumer. In lightly regulated states in the South and West, it is easier for young and healthy customers to find inexpensive plans that cover only major illnesses, but difficult for older people or those with even minor medical conditions to find coverage. In Texas, for instance, insurers are able to charge higher-risk people as much as 25 times more than healthy ones, and can raise rates for their plans based on a long list of preexisting conditions, from anxiety to acid reflux.

The new law seeks to rationalize this jumble with a clear set of rules. These rules apply primarily to people in the individual insurance market, because those covered by large employers already are protected against many controversial practices. Several of the rules will take effect this year. Others will begin in 2014 as part of the creation of the state-based "exchanges" where small businesses and people without employer-based insurance will be able to buy coverage.

insurers that institute unjustifiably high rate increases in the next few years from joining the exchanges when they open in 2014.

Analysts say that insurers may ultimately be constrained by another dynamic: competition. The industry is still exempt from antitrust laws. (While the House has passed a separate bill that would revoke that benefit, its fate in the Senate remains unclear.) But if the exchanges work as planned, they will offer consumers more options than are available now on the individual market. And if insurers are too aggressive with their rates in the first few years, they may lose out to lower-priced rivals.

"They're free to price themselves into oblivion if they choose to do so," says Sheryl Skolnick, an industry analyst with CRT Capital Group.

Temporary Solution for Preexisting Conditions

The biggest challenge before 2014 will be making insurance available to adults who have preexisting conditions, because rules guaranteeing them coverage will not take effect until January 2014. The law's temporary solution is to set aside $5 billion to pay for a federal high-risk pool where people with preexisting conditions could get coverage if they have been uninsured for six months. (See Chapter 1 for more about the pools.)

The Rules in the Exchanges

The new universe of regulations will arrive in full with the debut in 2014 of the exchanges on which people without employer-based insurance and small businesses will be able to buy coverage. In these new state-based marketplaces:

- Insurers will no longer be able to deny coverage to adults with preexisting conditions or charge them exorbitant rates.
- Insurers will be able to vary their rates, but only within strict limits: They will be able to charge older people three times more than younger ones (a far lower ratio than currently exists in many states) and will be able to charge smokers 1½ times as much as nonsmokers. The thinking is that insurers will be able to abide by these restrictions and still make a profit, because they will be enrolling many more young and healthy customers than they do now, as a result of the individual insurance mandate. Certain insurers may end up with a much higher-risk population than others, but the law calls for "risk adjustment," in which insurers with lower-risk enrollees must compensate the others.
- Insurers also will face new rules regarding the quality of

their plans. The health and human services secretary will determine a package of "essential benefits" the plans need to offer that will be equivalent to a typical employer-based plan. That package will spell out rough standards in a range of areas, such as maternity care, mental health treatment and emergency services. The plans must pay for at least 60 percent of the care people receive, with out-of-pocket costs limited to $5,950 for individuals and $11,900 for families (in 2010 dollars). Plans at this minimum level will receive a "bronze" rating. Insurers also can offer a "silver" plan that covers 70 percent of costs, a "gold" plan that covers 80 percent, and a "platinum" plan that covers 90 percent. They can offer low-priced plans with only catastrophic coverage to people younger than 30. (See Chapter 2 on the individual mandate.)

- Insurers will still be able to sell individual policies outside the exchanges, but buyers there will not receive government subsidies, and the plans will need to comply with the new rules pertaining to preexisting conditions and differences in premium rates. Plans off the exchanges could appeal to illegal immigrants, who are not allowed to buy through them, and potentially also to high-income people who do not qualify for the government subsidies and might be drawn to a non-exchange plan that offers better rates. Some experts worry that such plans could lure healthy people out of the exchanges, leaving a more costly pool of consumers.

Ban on Annual Limits

In addition to the ban on lifetime limits for benefits, in 2014 insurers both in and off the exchanges will face a ban on annual limits for benefits paid out. Even before 2014, the health and human services secretary will be able to set restrictions on annual benefits limits. Like the ban on lifetime limits, this rule will depend partly on how it is spelled out and enforced. Insurers may be able to find ways around it by limiting not dollar amounts but treatment for a given condition.

More Transparency

One of the biggest challenges for people who buy insurance on the individual market is finding out what they're actually getting for their money—and then knowing what to do if a claim is not covered. The exchanges are supposed to solve those problems, too. Insurers will need to report, in plain language, extensive information about their plans: procedures for paying claims, the number of claims denied, cost-sharing requirements and rules regarding out-of-network providers, among other details.

The states running the exchanges will be required to adopt several consumer-friendly practices, as well. They will have to maintain a customer service call center and establish clear procedures for enrolling people and determining eligibility for the subsidies, which will be transferred directly from the federal government to the insurer.

Will It Work?

The effectiveness of the new insurance rules will depend on regulators' ability—and willingness—to enforce them. The exchanges will be run by individual states, or possibly by groups of neighboring states. Given that many states currently have scant insurance regulations and are governed by leaders who oppose the new legislation, it is possible that exchanges in these states will fail to carry out the letter of the law. On the other hand, if people see the exchanges in other states become well-functioning marketplaces with strong consumer protections, there may be pressure to improve their own states' exchanges.

— Alec MacGillis

CHAPTER 4

The Insured:
It's Status Quo—For Now

As transformational as the new health-care law is, it will have relatively little impact, at least in the near future, on the majority of Americans who have employer-based insurance.

Short-Term Changes

Two rules that will take effect in September 2010 will benefit people who are covered by their employers:

1) Many parents will be able to keep their children on their policies until their 26th birthday, as long as those children are not offered coverage at their own jobs.
2) Insurers will no longer be able to limit lifetime benefits, a practice that is common in individual policies and increasingly prevalent in employer-based plans: Fifty-five percent of workers with employer-based coverage had a lifetime limit in 2007, including 23 percent with a cap of less than $2 million.

What the Law's Longer Term Impact May Be

If the law succeeds in slowing the growth of health-care costs, it could curb increases in premiums for employer-based coverage, which have more than doubled over the past decade. As premiums have increased, employers have responded by raising the employees' share, and by shifting to plans with higher deductibles and co-pays. Many economists also see a strong correlation between the rise in premiums and the stagnation in wages, as employers make up for higher health-care costs by limiting pay.

The only neutral arbiter to have ventured an informed estimate of future premium rates is the Congressional Budget Office. It predicted in 2009 that by 2016, the law would leave premiums for those with employer-based coverage somewhere between unchanged from where they would be without reform to about 3 percent lower. Proponents of the law noted, though, that the CBO was unable to calculate the effect of some measures, such as better use of electronic medical records and changes in the way care is delivered. If providers are able to reduce the growth in health-care costs by just 1.5 percent each year—the goal hospitals set as part of an agreement with the White House in 2009—the average premium for a family would be $3,700 lower by 2020 than it would be otherwise.

Skeptics doubt that the law will slow the growth of employer-based premiums. And they worry that the expansion of the Medicaid program will cause providers to charge private plans more to compensate for what they view as under-reimbursement by public plans.

A New Tax on High-Priced Plans

The new tax on high-priced insurance, or "Cadillac" plans, could lower premiums for employer-based coverage—and probably also result in higher out-of-pocket costs. Proponents say the tax is a way to raise revenue to pay for broader coverage, as well as a way to slow spending. It would do so by encouraging employers and employees to adopt plans with lower premiums. The idea is to make people with very generous insurance more sensitive to medical costs—either by raising the out-of-pocket costs for the plans,

WHY THE NEW LAW DOESN'T FOCUS ON EMPLOYER-BASED COVERAGE

Fifty-nine percent of all Americans have insurance through their employers, down from a high of 64 percent in 2000. But even as it shrinks, the system of employer-provided coverage remains, for now, the foundation of health-care financing in this country.

The employer-based system has its critics: Many argue, for one, that it is unfair that, because of a quirk of history, such benefits are exempt from income taxes, whereas people who buy their own coverage must do so with after-tax money. Not to mention that most workers have little or no choice of plans, and that it's left to companies to shoulder the administrative burdens of buying health insurance for their workers.

That said, most people in the employer-based system are protected from the most controversial insurance practices, such as being denied coverage for preexisting conditions or having their insurance revoked once they become sick. And many of them profess to be satisfied with their plans. So, to avoid upending too much of the system, the lawmakers who wrote the new legislation focused on the people who are worst off: the more than 45 million people without coverage; the 18 million who buy insurance on the individual market where prices tend to be high and regulations lax; and small businesses.

If the law works as intended, creating a well-functioning new marketplace where people can buy coverage on their own, it will set in motion a shift away from employer-based coverage. But it will be a gradual one.

or by encouraging them to switch to HMO-style plans such as Kaiser Permanente.

The tax was scaled back sharply amid concerns that it would hit many plans that are not particularly lavish but are expensive because they are offered in high-cost areas or by businesses with many older workers. Under the law, a 40 percent excise tax will be applied starting in 2018 to premiums in excess of $27,500 for families and $10,200 for individuals. As it now stands, only a tiny fraction of plans exceed these thresholds—the average family premium is $13,375 and the average individual premium is $4,824— but more plans are expected to cross as time goes on. The thresholds will increase at the rate of inflation, while premiums are expected to rise faster than that unless employers switch to less expensive plans.

The CBO predicts that if there is a shift to lower-cost plans, the government would still be collecting more tax revenue, because employers would pay out in higher wages some of the savings they gained from spending less on health insurance. But some economists doubt that wages will go up as a result of a shift to lower-priced plans; if the job market remains as slack as it is today, employers may not feel the need to raise wages to compete for workers.

Can I Use the Exchange?

For most people, having employer-based insurance is preferable to having to buy coverage on the individual market—after all, the employer pays for part of the premiums; and, unlike on the individual market, the premiums are paid on a pre-tax basis.

But some people with employer-based coverage may wish to take part in the new state-based exchanges that will be set up in 2014 for small businesses and people buying insurance on their own. People in the exchanges will still buy with after-tax dollars, but they'll qualify for income-based subsidies to help them afford coverage if they earn less than 400 percent of the poverty level, or $88,000 for a family of four. And if the exchanges work, they will offer a far broader range of choices than those available to people covered by their employers.

To keep the employer-based insurance system from unraveling, the law makes the exchanges off-limits, at least for now, to most people with coverage through their jobs. The only people who will be able to break from their employer plans to buy insurance on the exchanges will be those whose employers offer them inferior coverage—plans whose premiums cost employees more than 9.5 percent of their income or that fall beneath the minimum standard of insurance laid out by the law, covering less than 60 percent of medical costs and requiring very high out-of-pocket spending. These workers will be eligible for subsidies on the exchanges, and their employers will be penalized for offering poor coverage. In addition, workers whose incomes are below 400 percent of the poverty level and whose employer coverage costs them 8 percent to 9.8 percent of their pay can request a voucher from their employer, equal to the amount the employer was spending on their coverage, and use it to buy insurance on the exchange.

The other people with employer-based insurance who will be able to obtain coverage on the exchanges at the outset are those who work for businesses with fewer than 100 employees. But these workers will not receive the income-based subsidies that individuals buying on the exchanges will, because their employers will still be paying the bulk of the premiums.

Starting in 2017, employers with more than 100 workers will be able to buy coverage for them on the exchanges as well. How many choose to do so will depend on how well the exchanges are functioning.

Meanwhile, some employers that now offer coverage may decide to drop it and have their workers buy their own insurance on the exchanges, with the benefit of the income-based subsidies. Employers with more than 50 workers will have to pay a fine of $2,000 per worker if they do not provide coverage, which is less than most now pay for medical benefits. Health-care experts predict that relatively few employers will take this step at the outset, because the exchanges will be such an unknown that employers will still have a competitive hiring advantage if they offer benefits.

But if the exchanges flourish, they could become the new underlying structure for American health insurance. That would be a big change for many workers. But if employers make up their saved health-benefit costs in the form of higher wages, and if

WHAT ABOUT COBRA?

In 2014, the new insurance exchanges will effectively replace the Consolidated Omnibus Budget Reconciliation Act, commonly referred to as COBRA, the program that allows people to stay on their employer's plan for up to 18 months after they're laid off or leave their job, although at a steep price—an average of $1,100 per month for a family. The exchanges will provide the same guarantee of coverage even for people who have a preexisting condition. And if they work as planned, the exchanges will have premiums that are more affordable than COBRA's, particularly for those who qualify for subsidies.

Congress is still considering whether to renew the 65 percent COBRA subsidy that was included in the 2009 economic stimulus package, which reduced the average family premium to about $385 per month. That subsidy, which can be used for up to 15 months of COBRA coverage, expired on March 31, 2010, meaning that people laid off after that date must pay the full COBRA rate.

subsidies on the exchanges continue to keep plans there affordable, many workers may come to prefer the greater breadth of choices the exchanges offer.

Other Groups That Have Coverage

Veterans and the military

The law has no direct effect on the Veterans Affairs or Tricare system for military families. The VA received a 16 percent budget increase for the 2010 fiscal year, its largest increase in more than 30 years, followed by an administration request for a 7.6 percent increase for next year.

Native Americans

The law includes a permanent reauthorization of the Indian Health Care Improvement Act, which lapsed in 2001. This will bring with it a 13 percent budget increase for the Indian Health Service.

Federal employees

Most federal workers will continue to receive coverage through the Federal Employees Health Benefits Program administered by the Office of Personnel Management. But Congress members and their staffs will be required to obtain coverage on the state-based exchanges.

People satisfied with their individual plan

Many people with individual coverage are likely to switch to the exchanges, where there will be more choices and clearer rules, as well as subsidies available to most consumers. Some may wish to stick with their existing individual plans, particularly if they earn too much to qualify for the subsidies. Insurers will be permitted to offer individual plans outside of the exchanges, but whether they continue to do so will depend on how the market shapes up in 2014, as millions of individual customers shift to the exchanges.

— *Alec MacGillis*

CHAPTER 5

Under Thirty:
Joining the System, Like It or Not

Once the bill's main provisions are fully phased in by 2014, more than 95 percent of children will be eligible for coverage, and the largest group of uninsured individuals—young adults in their 20s—will have access to more affordable insurance options than the limited number of policies that exist today on the individual market.

Short-Term Benefits

Four provisions related to children and young adults will take effect in September 2010:

1) Insurance companies may not deny coverage to children who have preexisting conditions. (To learn about the controversy over this provision, see Chapter 3.)
2) Adult children may be enrolled in their parents' insurance plans until they turn 26, provided they do not receive coverage through their own employers.
3) Most health-care plans will be required to provide immunizations, physicals and other preventive care for infants and children, without co-pays, deductibles or other cost-sharing fees.

4) However serious their budget problems, states will be barred from limiting children's eligibility for Medicaid or the Children's Health Insurance Program, known as CHIP, which together provide coverage for more than 30 million low-income children.

Benefits and Changes That Phase in Over a Longer Period

Over the first five years, Medicaid and CHIP will be retooled:

1) Starting in 2014, the Medicaid program, which is run jointly with states and varies widely in eligibility and enrollment requirements, will be streamlined to guarantee coverage to all Americans with incomes below 133 percent of the federal poverty level, regardless of where they live. Currently, children younger than 6 are covered by Medicaid if their household incomes fall under the 133 percent threshold. But 27 states cut off eligibility at 100 percent for children ages 6 to 18.

2) The CHIP program, which also is run jointly with states, mainly serves children and pregnant women who live above the poverty level but who can't afford private insurance. The law says the program must continue until at least 2019, though it leaves its funding somewhat in doubt. It allocates federal funding only until 2015. But at the same time, the law says that, starting in 2015, the federal government will pick up a greater share of the program's costs.

In other words, the law does not spell out whether states must continue to provide coverage through CHIP after 2015, or whether eligible children will be shifted—along with their parents—to the new state insurance exchanges, where they could buy coverage with the help of subsidies. The law does say that children may not be moved out of CHIP until they are guaranteed at least the same benefits elsewhere.

3) In addition to having the opportunity to remain on their parents' plans until their 26th birthday, young adults up to age 30 will have the additional option of buying less expensive plans that cover catastrophic conditions on the state exchanges once they begin operating in 2014. These plans will be offered to individuals up to age 30 and would cover only major medical expenses, with the exception of three primary-care visits per year that would be exempt from the deductible.

Broader Questions and Potential Unintended Consequences

What about the children of illegal immigrants?

According to the Pew Hispanic Center, about 700,000 children who are classified as illegal immigrants do not have health-care coverage. Under the new law, they—along with their parents—will be ineligible for Medicaid and CHIP as well as for coverage offered through exchanges. The new law preserves the current five-year waiting period for documented immigrants to enroll in Medicaid after achieving legal status.

Will Medicaid, CHIP and the exchanges have the same eligibility requirements?

Health-care experts worry that Medicaid, CHIP and the exchanges will require conflicting forms of documentation and other enrollment procedures, leading to confusion among low-income families and potentially reducing the likelihood that they will seek coverage.

For instance, to determine a child's eligibility for CHIP, states are permitted to set their own rules for establishing household income, often relying on pay stubs and records of child-support payments. Under the new law, eligibility for subsidies on the state exchanges will be determined by federal tax returns.

When Congress reauthorized the CHIP program in 2009, it added incentives for states to simplify enrollment procedures. But the process is expected to become more complex once the state exchanges are operating.

An estimated 8 million Americans are eligible for Medicaid under the current system, but have not enrolled. Although Medicaid eligibility rules will be simplified, determining efficient ways to move low-income people, including children, off the uninsured rolls and into the appropriate federal health-care assistance program is a challenge. Health-care experts are particularly concerned about this problem in the South, where Medicaid coverage is currently minimal.

Another challenge is moving young adults from CHIP to the exchanges once they turn 19 and no longer qualify for that public program. It remains unclear how long this challenge will exist, because, after several years, states will be allowed to eliminate CHIP and simply enroll everyone who would have qualified for it into an exchange, or possibly Medicaid, instead.

The new law does include provisions aimed at further streamlining enrollment, with the long-term goal of creating a single point of entry for individuals and families that are eligible for federal aid—be it Medicaid, CHIP, or subsidies for private coverage on the exchanges.

Will it get easier to find a pediatrician who accepts Medicaid?

Medicaid reimburses physicians at far lower rates than Medicare, resulting in chronic shortages of doctors willing to treat Medicaid patients, including children. The new law will lift Medicaid payment rates to Medicare levels beginning in 2013 for primary care, including pediatrics, to encourage more doctors to participate.

Will I still be able to take my child to our local community health center?

Yes. The nation's network of 1,250 federally supported primary-care clinics will get a huge boost in funding under the new law: $11 billion over five years. Children of illegal immigrants may use them.

Why are catastrophic policies available only to individuals younger than 30?

In health-care parlance, people in their 20s are the "young invincibles." Because they are mostly healthy and often work part-time or for employers that don't offer coverage, they have the highest uninsured rate of any age group, constituting about 30 percent of the overall population without coverage.

Their absence deprives insurance pools of healthy people to help balance out the cost of sicker policyholders. The new insurance mandate will require young adults to buy coverage or face a fine, but lawmakers were wary about imposing too large a financial burden on young people and decided to create a special catastrophic plan that would cost less than other packages offered on the exchanges (See Chapters 1 and 2).

Some economists view the catastrophic plan as a gateway to an intriguing new coverage model, in which doctor visits and routine treatment would be paid for out of pocket by patients, and insurance would be reserved for the largest costs.

— Shailagh Murray

CHAPTER 6

The Medicare Changes: Dollars and Doughnuts

Americans age 65 and older are not a main focus of the new health-care law, because they are already insured under Medicare, the federal program that brings that group a lot closer to universal coverage than any other age category. Even so, the law makes several important changes that will affect many of the 46 million people Medicare serves.

Among the most significant: The government will provide more help with paying for prescription drugs, although not all at once. Over the next 10 years, a gap in prescription drug coverage—called the "doughnut hole," because there is coverage below and above the gap—will shrink gradually until it disappears. This eventually will save as much as a few thousand dollars a year for older Americans who take a lot of higher-priced medications.

A second change, which is not friendly to consumers, is designed to save the government money. The change affects Medicare recipients who belong to private managed-care plans, instead of the traditional fee-for-service version of the program. The government will reduce the amount of money it pays to the private plans that cover people through a part of the program known as Medicare Advantage. The private plans, not patients, will take the direct hit.

But the plans may, in turn, charge consumers more, reduce benefits or drop out of some communities altogether.

Both of these changes complete a political boomerang. Seven years ago, the then-Republican majority in Congress created the drug benefits and the Medicare Advantage payment rates. Democrats have been waiting ever since to redesign them.

Two other noteworthy changes for beneficiaries:

- Older Americans will pay less for preventive care.
- For the first time, affluent people will pay more than others for Medicare's drug coverage. Also, more people with higher incomes will have to pay extra in premiums for doctor visits and other services outside a hospital.

Now, the specifics.

Better Drug Benefits

Medicare used to differ from almost all other health insurance plans because it did not offer a prescription drug benefit. Then in 2003, Congress created such a benefit, known as Medicare Part D.

Part D became available in 2006 and quickly proved popular. About 34 million people—nearly 75 percent of everyone in Medicare—have Part D coverage today. But until now, the drug benefit has contained a highly unpopular quirk: Because the lawmakers who created it wanted to limit the government's cost, they designed it with an unusual gap in coverage, the infamous doughnut hole. That gap has required people who use a lot of higher-priced medications to shoulder much of the cost themselves—up to $3,610 in 2010—even as they continued to be responsible for paying their Part D premium. About one in seven people with Medicare drug coverage fell into the doughnut hole during 2007, the most recent year for which data are available.

The new coverage will work the same way the prescription benefit always did, before the gap kicked in: Beneficiaries first will pay a deductible (unless they're insured through one of the private health plans that picks up the deductible cost). After that, Medicare covers 75 percent of drug expenses, leaving consumers responsible for up to 25 percent.

Only a few people are expected to reach the high "catastrophic" threshold, estimated to be nearly $13,000 in 2020 in total spending, according to the Medicare Actuary, an office in the Health and Human Services Department's Centers for Medicare and Medicaid Services. Total spending means the combination of what Medicare covers and what consumers pay (the deductible, the 25 percent before the gap and all costs inside the gap).

The law will set in motion a complicated, phased-in process to fill the doughnut hole, which will narrow and then close permanently in 2020. (See chart on following page for how the phase-in will work.) At that time, people will have the same 75 percent level of coverage until they reach the catastrophic threshold. Beyond that, Medicare will pick up 95 percent of the rest.

The rules are different for brand-name drugs and lower-priced generics:

Brand-name drugs. A little help will begin right away: The government will give a $250 rebate in 2010 to anyone who falls in the gap. The current threshold for reaching the gap is $2,830.

More assistance will arrive in 2011. From then on, much of the help will come from the pharmaceutical industry. Manufacturers of brand-name drugs will be required to provide 50 percent discounts to people once they enter the doughnut hole. The law does not place any restrictions on the prices that drug manufacturers may charge; they are simply required to cut that price in half.

Then, in 2013, the government also will provide a subsidy, which will start small and increase gradually until 2020. By that year, the 50 percent discount from the manufacturers, combined with a 25 percent government subsidy, will cover 75 percent of a person's drug expenses. At that point, all Medicare beneficiaries will have the same level of coverage, no matter how much they

Filling the Doughnut Hole

The new law eventually will eliminate a gap in coverage, or doughnut hole, that affects about one in seven people who have Medicare drug benefits.

Under the old law

After a deductible — $310 in 2010 — not covered by the government, Part D has three stages:

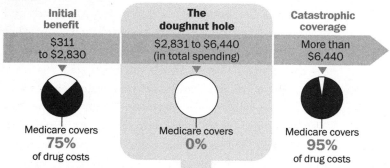

Initial benefit	The doughnut hole	Catastrophic coverage
$311 to $2,830	$2,831 to $6,440 (in total spending)	More than $6,440
Medicare covers **75%** of drug costs	Medicare covers **0%**	Medicare covers **95%** of drug costs

Under the new law

The gap will shrink slowly at first, then accelerate until it disappears in 2020. The additional coverage will be phased in separately for brand-name drugs and generics.

	BRAND-NAME DRUG COVERAGE			GENERIC COVERAGE
	Discount from drugmakers +	Part D benefit =	Total % covered	Part D benefit, % covered
2010*	0%	0%	0%	0%
2011	50	0	50	7
2012	50	0	50	14
2013	50	2.5	52.5	21
2014	50	2.5	52.5	28
2015	50	5	55	35
2016	50	5	55	42
2017	50	10	60	49
2018	50	15	65	56
2019	50	20	70	63
2020	50	25	75	75

*In 2010, Medicare will give those who reach the doughnut hole a **one-time $250 rebate**.

SOURCE: Centers for Medicare and Medicaid Services

spend on drugs—except for those few who reach the catastrophic level.

Generic drugs. This part is more straightforward. Starting in 2011, the government will gradually increase the benefit for generic drugs after people reach the coverage gap. The program will start by paying for an extra 7 percent, and then will phase in more help until it is covering 75 percent by 2020. Again, the gap will be closed and people will pay 25 percent of the expense for their medicine.

For the moment, the best experts in Congress, in the Medicare Actuary's office and in the health policy world outside government say they have not calculated exactly what these two kinds of help will provide in dollars and cents. They say it is hard to predict the mix of brand-name drugs and generics that a given patient is likely to use.

A small twist for retirees

The law could create a disruption for retirees who receive prescription drug coverage through their former employers. They could lose that benefit, because starting in 2013, the law will prevent companies from deducting from their taxes a $1,330 per-person subsidy that employers have been receiving under the 2003 law that created Part D.

Once that subsidy is no longer tax-deductible, some employers may stop offering the benefit to retirees, who presumably would switch to Medicare's drug coverage instead.

Less Advantage to Medicare Advantage

The law contains a big reversal when it comes to the private health plans in Medicare. When Republicans controlled Congress and the White House, they were eager to encourage older Americans to sign up for managed-care plans. They renamed this part of the program Medicare Advantage. And they decided to pay these insurers more money, in hope that the companies would, in turn, offer inducements for Medicare patients to join.

Democrats, however, have always had a different view, believing the government was overpaying. The new law reflects that view. The change will start in 2011, when Medicare's payments will freeze at the 2010 level. After that, the rates will decrease over three to six years, depending on the location.

In the end, Medicare's payments to private health plans will decrease on average by about 12 percent, saving the government an estimated $132 billion over the coming decade. Exactly how much less money will go to the plans will vary from county to county, under a complicated formula that takes into account the cost of health care in each place and how much the insurers receive now, compared with the local rates in the traditional version of Medicare. Under a four-tier system, the plans will end up being paid 95 percent to 115 percent of the fee-for-service rates in the counties they serve.

This payment change could matter a lot to patients. The reason? The plans are not likely to absorb the cuts. They probably will do something to recoup the money they lose. No one can say in advance exactly how; congressional budget analysts estimate that nearly 5 million fewer people in Medicare will have private health plans in 2019 than if the law had not changed.

In the meantime, a few experts have begun trying to predict the consequences. An analysis by Brian Biles, a George Washington University professor who has worked on health policy in and out of the government, suggests that about two-thirds of the plans will end up being paid less than the local cost of caring for Medicare patients. He and Marsha Gold, a think-tank analyst who has specialized in managed-care Medicaid, predict that, although some plans will drop out of the program, more are likely to cut back on services such as vision care, or enhanced coverage for drugs or hospital stays.

In other words, once the cuts have taken place and the plans

PRIVATE HEALTH PLANS IN MEDICARE: GROWTH AND CONTROVERSY

Being enrolled in a private managed-care plan is very different from taking part in the traditional version of Medicare, in which patients choose any doctor or other provider of care and the government pays on a fee-for-service basis. These private plans, now known collectively as Medicare Advantage, have been part of Medicare for years. Congress began to encourage them more through the Balanced Budget Agreement of 1997, as part of an effort to save money.

But in 2006, the government started to pay the plans more generously, triggering a growth spurt as more insurers decided to sign up. Since then, the number of health plans that accept Medicare patients has more than tripled, to nearly 3,000. The result? About a quarter of people on Medicare today participate in a private plan.

All this growth sparked a controversy. Many Medicare policy experts have contended that these private plans have been getting paid too much; nationwide, the government pays them, on average, 113 percent of the regular Medicare rates for doctors, hospitals and others. The insurance industry has countered that those payments are legitimate and have been good for patients. Some plans have used the money to offer drug coverage without premiums, as well as extra benefits, such as vision care and gym memberships, that Medicare traditionally has not covered.

have responded, older Americans will have to decide whether managed care is a good deal for them.

People of Means

The law expands on a recent and controversial aspect of Medicare in which wealthier older Americans must pay higher premiums. The idea is known as a "means test," or an income-related premium. Exactly how much more someone pays depends on his or her income. After years of political debate, means-testing became a reality in 2007 for Part B of the program, the portion that covers doctor's visits and other outpatient medical services. Why did Congress require those with higher incomes to pay extra? For the sole purpose of bringing more money into the program.

Under the law, means-testing will spread to Part D, the prescription drug benefit. At the same time, a subtle but important change in the Part B rules will, a decade from now, cause an estimated 1 million more people to pay higher premiums for that part of the program.

Here is how this will work:

Premiums for drug coverage (Part D). Starting in January 2011, Part D will adopt the same means test being used for Part B. Single people with incomes of $85,000 or higher, and couples with incomes of $170,000 or higher, will have to pay larger premiums for coverage. The higher their income, the larger the surcharge, with four escalating levels. The Medicare Actuary predicts that this change will affect an estimated 1.4 million people—about 1.1 million will pay a higher premium, while perhaps 300,000 will drop their coverage rather than pay more for it.

Part B premiums. When Medicare began to means-test this part of the program, the idea was that the surcharges would apply to about 5 percent of the people with such coverage. To prevent that percentage from rising, the income threshold has gone up each year, keeping pace with inflation.

Here is the change: Starting in 2011 and lasting until 2019, the program will no longer "index"—or increase—the income threshold each year. The result? Because incomes tend to rise, the number of Medicare beneficiaries who will reach the threshold to pay more will creep upward annually. The Medicare Actuary predicts that by 2019, about 5.3 million in Medicare will have to pay extra for their premiums, compared with about 4.3 million if the law had not changed.

An Ounce of Prevention

The government is trying to motivate older Americans to seek preventive care, with the goal of warding off debilitating, costly illnesses. The law does this in a simple way. Starting in 2011, Medicare recipients will no longer have to pay anything out of pocket for a set of preventive services the program already covers, as long as they do not exceed Medicare's limits on each one. Those services include a physical, help with quitting smoking, and a variety of tests relating to cancer, cholesterol, bone density, diabetes and other medical issues.

—Amy Goldstein

CHAPTER 7

Long-Term Care: A New National Option

Although they have not received much attention, there are provisions in the legislation that address one of the country's most profound and anguishing issues: how and where we live when we are young and disabled or old and frail.

The law will make the biggest changes to the nation's system of long-term care since the creation of Medicaid in 1965. Chief among them are:

- a new voluntary, national long-term care insurance program and
- steps that will make Medicaid benefits more broadly available to those living at home.

The CLASS Act

The Community Living Assistance Services and Supports (CLASS) Act creates, for the first time, a national long-term care insurance system. By 2012 you should be able to buy a policy that will make you eligible for a basic lifetime cash benefit to help pay for care should you become disabled. The law sets only a broad framework for this insurance. Details, including premium levels and benefits, will be worked out over the next couple of years.

If I want to enroll, how will I do so?

Anybody over 18 will be eligible to enroll, as long as they have at least a part-time job. If your employer agrees to participate, you'll automatically be signed up for the insurance, although you'll be allowed to opt out. If your company does not offer the option, you'll be able to enroll directly through the government. As long as you are working you'll be able to buy insurance even if you already have health problems.

If you decide to opt out of the insurance initially, you'll be able to enroll later, but you'll pay a penalty: Premiums are tied to your age, so the longer you wait, the bigger the monthly payment you'll make.

How expensive will the premiums be?

Premiums must be set so the CLASS program will remain solvent for at least 75 years. To assure it remains sustainable, the government will be allowed to raise premiums if the program appears to be losing money.

Supporters hope premiums will average less than $100 a month. More than that, and they fear few people will buy. Worse, those who do are likely to be those most likely to need it, which will drive premiums higher still. If you are very poor or a student, you'll pay a discounted monthly premium that may be as little as $5.

What will benefits consist of?

The average benefit will be at least $50 a day. Once a doctor or other health provider certifies that you need care, you'll be covered for as long as necessary. And because the benefit will be in cash, you'll be able to use it to pay family members or friends for care or even renovate your home to make it, say, wheelchair accessible.

One caveat: You'll have to pay premiums for at least five years before you are eligible for benefits.

THE NEED FOR LONG-TERM CARE

More than 10 million Americans need long-term care, which is considered personal, rather than medical, assistance.

Long-term care may involve help with eating, bathing or going to the bathroom, or assistance with getting to the doctor or managing medications. More than 80 percent of people who receive this care live at home, and about 15 percent live in skilled nursing facilities.

Most long-term care services are provided by family members and friends, often at great financial, physical and emotional cost. At the same time, Americans spend more than $200 billion out of pocket every year for paid assistance from home-care aides, nursing facilities and other services.

Medicaid, the joint state and federal health-care program that was created primarily to provide medical treatment for young mothers and children, now pays for nearly half of all long-term care, at a cost of more than $100 billion, or one-third of its budget.

Medicare, the health program for seniors, pays for short-term nursing and home care, but it does not cover long-term care.

Medicaid is available only to those who are very poor and very sick. Middle-class people typically end up on Medicaid only after they have spent virtually all of their money on medical and long-term care.

About 7 million Americans have private long-term care insurance to help cover the costs.

*Will I be able to keep my private
long-term care insurance?*

Yes. In fact, some insurance companies may design policies to supplement CLASS coverage, much like Medigap does with basic Medicare. Others think they'll be able to sell policies to compete with the CLASS Act.

Will it work?

Although supporters of the program believe participation will be high, industry experts, as well as the Congressional Budget Office and the Medicare actuary, predict that fewer than 6 percent of adults will buy CLASS insurance. Some critics of the proposal argue that if this happens the program will change from a fully-funded insurance system to just another budget-busting government entitlement program. Another possibility is that Congress could someday change the program from voluntary insurance to mandatory coverage. That's how most other developed countries cover long-term care and, of course, similar to the way the United States will now provide health insurance. In the long run, a successful long-term care insurance system—whether government or private—would reduce the financial burden on Medicaid.

Broader Medicaid Benefits

For now, the Medicaid program will continue to be the biggest payer of long-term care services. But the new law also makes big changes in the way that the joint state-federal program helps those needing long-term care.

Today states are required to provide Medicaid long-term care only to those living in nursing homes. States are allowed to provide home-care benefits as well, as long as they receive the okay from the federal government. But most of these home-care programs are badly underfunded.

The new law will help states expand this assistance in two ways:

1) The federal government will pay states extra to encourage them to make more home-care services available to people who would otherwise be in nursing homes. It will also reduce the red tape that states must cut through to offer these programs.

2) The new law will also help families by allowing spouses of those who need long-term care to hang on to extra assets when care is delivered at home. Today couples must often spend nearly all of their assets before one spouse is eligible for community care.

In the face of severe budget problems, many states are cutting back on their home-care programs. As a result, the law's additional federal funding may not do much more than maintain minimal assistance for those who want to stay at home.

Better Coordination Between Medicaid and Medicare

The law provides better coordinated care for those poorest and sickest who are eligible for both Medicaid and Medicare. It is not uncommon for these nearly eight million people to have five or more chronic diseases and be taking a dozen medications.

Because Medicare pays for health care and Medicaid provides personal care, it has always been a challenge to coordinate benefits. For instance, Medicare will pay tens of thousands of dollars to treat a heart attack, but won't provide the care that someone suffering from chronic heart disease needs to stay at home. And Medicaid may not pay for that home care either. As a result, patients often suffer needless hospitalizations that take a toll on their health and cost the government billions of dollars: Medicare typically spends twice as much on care for those who are enrolled in both programs as on other seniors.

The health law creates a Federal Coordinated Health Care office that will help Medicare and Medicaid manage treatment and care. This office will, among other steps, encourage new ways to deliver care to those receiving both Medicare and Medicaid benefits.

— Howard Gleckman

CHAPTER 8

Delivery of Care: Breaking Bad Habits

Most of the spending in the new health-care law—and the discussion around it—is focused on expanding coverage to 32 million people who would otherwise lack it. But many of the law's hundreds of pages are taken up with its equally ambitious goal of transforming how the nation's medical system provides care.

The theory behind most of the "delivery system" reforms is simple: American medical providers are too often rewarded for quantity of care rather than quality, which helps explain why the country spends so much more of its resources on health care than other developed nations while getting, in many instances, poorer outcomes.

The new law includes a wide array of measures intended to move away from this approach. The legislation does not rely on the hoped-for savings from these changes to pay for coverage of the uninsured; the Congressional Budget Office said it could not estimate the savings that most of the measures will produce. But it is these delivery-system changes that the administration is counting on to "bend the curve" of the nation's overall medical spending, both public and private, to keep health-care costs from devouring the economy.

WHY THE EMPHASIS ON QUANTITY, NOT QUALITY?

The heavy utilization of tests and treatments that has long characterized American medicine stems partly from the United States' the-more-the-better mentality—the kind of thinking that leads someone with a sports injury to insist on surgery, or that leads a man with elevated PSA levels to proceed with prostate removal instead of the "watchful waiting" that is more common in other developed countries.

It also results from the prevalence of the fee-for-service payment system, in which doctors and hospitals are paid for each test or procedure they perform, instead of receiving a lump sum to address a given condition or keep a certain person healthy. If, say, a hospital releases a man with heart disease and does not follow up to make sure he is taking proper care of himself, the odds are greater that he will need to be rehospitalized. But that hospital will be paid more for that readmission than another one that took the time for follow-ups for which it receives little reimbursement.

Changing Behavior From the Ground Up

For the most part, the law does not order medical providers to change how they do business, but instead creates incentives to prompt change from below. These incentives will be imbedded within Medicare and Medicaid, because those systems are under government purview, but the hope is that they will spark system-wide reforms that also will lower costs for private insurers.

The law creates pilot programs in both Medicare and Medicaid to develop "bundled" payments: In the Medicare pilot, a hospital would be paid a set amount for a period of care beginning three days before hospitalization and ending 30 days after discharge, giving the hospital an incentive to coordinate care in cost-effective ways. The law also creates a demonstration project that encourages providers to care for high-need Medicare patients at home, reducing the need for hospitalization. And it creates an "innovation center" within the Centers for Medicare and Medicaid Services to evaluate and expand payment structures that doctors and hospitals devise.

The law also encourages the spread of "accountable-care organizations"— networks of providers who agree to be responsible for the overall care of patients, and in which doctors typically are paid a salary rather than on a fee-for-service basis. This model is not unlike the "capitation" model that HMOs practiced in the 1990s, in which a network of providers was paid a set sum to care for a given person. But its proponents say more safeguards are in place to emphasize quality of care and discourage the corner-cutting or denial of care that the model could in theory spawn.

The accountable-care provision could end up complementing another provision in the law that allocates $6 billion in seed money for new member-owned nonprofit cooperative insurance plans. Accountable-care networks of providers could team up with new nonprofit insurance plans created for patients in their region; similar co-op systems that combine providers and insurers in one entity already exist in Seattle and Minneapolis.

"We're going to be effective by making health-care organizations responsible for the population's health," said Jeffrey E. Thompson, chief executive of Gundersen Lutheran, a hospital in LaCrosse, Wis., that uses the salaried, accountable-care model. "You make people responsible for the success of the organization—based not on how many surgeries they do, but the health of the population."

Some of the incentives for changing provider behavior are more blunt. Starting in 2012, Medicare payments will be reduced for hospitals with high levels of preventable readmissions—just one attempt to address the fact that nearly half of the country's health-care spending is used to treat the sickest 5 percent of the population. Also in 2012, Medicare will establish a value-based purchasing program in which hospitals will be paid more based on performance measures. Three years later, hospitals will be docked Medicare money for hospital-acquired infections. And, over the next few years, the government will implement a new payment formula for Medicare to reward doctors and hospitals for providing "high value" care—that is, hospitals that spend less per Medicare patient without reducing the quality of services.

This final provision already has sparked a fierce regional standoff: The hospitals with low per-patient spending that stand to receive more money under a new "value index" are clustered in the Upper Midwest and Pacific Northwest, while the high spenders who stand to lose out are concentrated in the South and in big cities such as Los Angeles, Miami and New York. The high-spending hospitals argue that they spend more partly because their more diverse patient populations have costlier conditions than the more homogenous populations in the lower-spending regions.

Changing Guidance From Above

There are also some more traditional top-down attempts to control spending. The law calls for a range of actions to clamp down on Medicare and Medicaid fraud. It creates an independent payment advisory board for Medicare—a 15-member panel that, starting in 2014, will submit to Congress recommendations to reduce the rate of Medicare spending. Congress can reject the suggestions only if it can come up with the same amount of reductions on its own or if it can muster 60 Senate votes to block the recommendations. It is modeled on the commission that recommends military base closures—taking politically difficult decisions out of lawmakers' hands.

The new legislation also creates a nonprofit institute to engage in comparative-effectiveness research, using data made possible by the spread of electronic medical records to research what treatments work best.

The law takes great pains to shield both of these entities from the accusation that they will resemble the "death panels" that the legislation's opponents said would be established. The Medicare

WHAT HAPPENED TO THE "DEATH PANELS"?

Former Alaska governor Sarah Palin evoked that scary phrase in the summer of 2009 to rally opposition to the health-care legislation. The former Republican presidential candidate used her Facebook page to dramatize a bogus interpretation of a provision in the original House bill that would have allowed Medicare reimbursement for physicians who provide end-of-life counseling. "The America I know and love is not one in which my parents or my baby with Down syndrome will have to stand in front of Obama's 'death panel,' " she wrote.

Hospitals and advocacy groups had pushed for the reimbursement clause, saying that doctors who take the time to help people craft "advance care directives" should get paid for it. Any counseling, proponents said, would be done on a strictly voluntary basis.

Palin's reply: "Is it any wonder that senior citizens might view such consultations as attempts to convince them to help reduce health-care costs by accepting minimal end-of-life care?"

After the furor subsided, the House kept the provision in the bill it approved. But the Senate left it out of its measure, and that version became the new law. Those seeking Medicare payment for end-of-life counseling say they will try again in the future.

commission is prohibited from making proposals that would ration care or change benefits, eligibility or cost-sharing for Medicare patients; and the law delays the panel's power to even address hospital rates until 2019. The comparative-effectiveness findings, meanwhile, may not be construed as mandates to guide payment and coverage decisions. One senior administration official acknowledged that while research may point to wasteful practices, the reform would for the time being not ask the "harder question" of what to do "if new technology does work better and reduces risks but costs a lot more, and how to evaluate that."

Will It Work?

There are grounds for skepticism. The political pressures these efforts will run into are foreshadowed by the limits placed on the Medicare commission and on comparative effectiveness. A vigorous debate continues about whether the regional differences in spending really are a sign of waste in some areas, and those that stand to lose out under the new formulas will not give up easily.

It remains to be seen whether bundled payments and accountable-care organizations will be able to avoid the controversies that HMOs encountered in trying to make care more efficient. There is also a concern that the spread of accountable-care organizations, while encouraging more coordinated and efficient care in many areas, could also end up creating medical monopolies that would increase provider prices. The law does much to try to reduce the use of medical care. But it does little to control the prices that doctors, hospitals, and drug and device makers charge, as a new government-run insurance plan, or "public option," might have done.

— Alec MacGillis

CHAPTER 9

On the Front Lines:
How Medical Practice Will Change

In many respects, American doctors today labor much the way their counterparts did 50 years ago.

Most are in practices with five or fewer other physicians. They keep their records on paper in longhand. When they need to consult a colleague, they reach for the telephone. They bill for each visit. They have little idea about how their skills compare to those of fellow practitioners, nor do most know what their patients really think about the care they give.

The new health-care law aims to change most of that.

Team Medicine

Fifty years from now, it is likely that most doctors will be members of teams that include case managers, social workers, dietitians, telephone counselors, data crunchers, guideline instructors, performance evaluators and external reviewers. They will be parts of organizations (which either employ them or contract with them) that are responsible for patients in and out of the hospital, in sickness and in health, over decades.

The records of what they do—and what every other doctor does—for a patient will be in electronic form, accessible from any computer. The software will gently remind them what to consider as they treat, and try to prevent, diseases. How the patients fare will be measured and publicized, and used in part to judge practitioners' performance. At the same time, the organizations, aided by the government, will make an effort to let caregivers know the "best practices" they're expected to follow.

These edifices, with primary care as the chief structural support, go by names such as "accountable care organizations" and "patient-centered medical homes." Some health-care systems, including Kaiser Permanente, Group Health Cooperative and the Mayo Clinic, already have versions of them.

Some physicians resent the fact that the new law promotes this evolutionary change. Others think it is liberating.

But one thing is clear: There are a lot of unhappy people practicing medicine right now.

A survey of physicians in 119 clinics in New York and the Midwest published in the Annals of Internal Medicine in 2009 found that 48 percent reported working in "chaotic" environments. Thirty percent said they needed at least half again more time for appointments as they were given. Only one-quarter said their practices strongly emphasized quality. Nearly one-third said they were likely to leave their jobs in the next two years.

If the new types of practice envisioned by the Patient Protection and Affordable Care Act take hold, much of that could change for the better.

"We are getting reports that patients are happy, physicians are happy and that, in at least some cases, they are saving money," said J. Fred Ralston Jr., president of the American College of Physicians. "It appears that when a doctor happens to be in a place that moves to a 'medical home' model, they can turn their frustration into excitement again. That is huge."

Ralston's practice, made up of eight physicians in Fayetteville, Tenn. (pop. 7,166), is too small to make the transition. He's a little bit sorry.

IN MASSACHUSETTS, SATISFIED DOCTORS

As provisions in the health-care law take effect in the next few years, most doctors will like them, although many won't feel much difference in their professional lives.

At least that's what the experience in Massachusetts suggests.

Massachusetts enacted near-universal health coverage in 2006. By the spring of 2009, only 2.7 percent of its residents were uninsured, an achievement unequaled in the 49 other states.

"Getting everybody covered in the state was just extraordinarily popular. I think that will show up on a national level, too," said Robert J. Blendon of the Harvard School of Public Health, whose research team conducted a poll of 2,135 Massachusetts physicians in late 2009.

The survey found that 70 percent of the doctors supported the health-care law. Thirteen percent opposed it, and 7 percent wanted it repealed. Half said it was reducing the number of uninsured patients they saw. One-third said they experienced increased "administrative burdens." Nearly two-thirds said it had "not much of an impact" on their personal financial situation.

One-third also said the reform law improved the quality of medical care in the state. One-third said it was "hurting" patients' ability to see a primary-care provider (with a slightly smaller fraction saying the opposite, that it was "helping"). Half the respondents said it was increasing the overall cost of care in the state.

Emphasis on Primary Care

In addition to extending health insurance to nearly all Americans, the new law seeks to raise the quality of medical practice, improve health in a measurable way, reduce waste and duplication, prevent medical error, enhance patient safety, and—hardest of all—"bend the curve" of rising costs.

Key to all those goals is primary care. Through many routes, the law provides a total of $26.4 billion over ten years to support this broad field of medicine, which, dozens of studies have shown, improves health and controls costs.

States with a higher per-capita ratio of primary-care physicians have lower mortality rates from cancer, heart disease and stroke. Having one additional primary-care physician in an underserved area is associated with 1.44 fewer premature deaths per 10,000 people. It also reduces spending per Medicare patient by $684. In 2000, 5 million hospital admissions, costing a total of $26.5 billion, might have been prevented with better primary care, according to one analysis.

A doctor shortage

The trouble is that there aren't enough primary-care physicians, and a declining fraction of new medical school graduates want to become them.

By 2025, there will be a shortage of 35,000 to 44,000 primary-care physicians in the United States, according to a recent estimate. (The country has about 661,000 practicing physicians and surgeons.) With the growth and aging of the population, the workload of primary-care doctors will increase by 29 percent over that period, too. From 1997 to 2005, the number of medical school graduates choosing family medicine fell by half. In 2007, only 23 percent of internal medicine residents planned to enter primary care, down from 54 percent a decade earlier.

The new law has several provisions designed to make primary care more attractive. It increases Medicare reimbursement for "evaluation and management" services—the government's name for examining and talking to the patient. It provides about $350 million in additional support for training programs in primary care. It sets a policy that hospital residency "slots" (largely paid for by Medicare) that go unfilled will be redistributed to programs that produce primary-care doctors. It provides loan-forgiveness incentives to medical school graduates who practice primary care in underserved areas.

Help from nurses

Nurses and physician assistants (PAs) also practice primary care, and the new law aims to increase their contribution, too.

Of 3.1 million registered nurses in the country, 158,000 are nurse practitioners working in primary care. Of 74,000 PAs, 26,000 are in primary care. The law states that both professions are essential to solving the nation's health-care problems. PA training programs with a history of producing graduates who go into primary care will be eligible for grants. There will be student loan debt forgiveness for nurses who go into teaching, which will help produce more nurse practitioners. The legislation pays for more school nurses, which experts hope will lead to healthier habits for children. A demonstration project testing whether chronically ill people can be cared for entirely in their homes uses nurse practitioners.

Nurse practitioners ($82,000) and primary-care PAs ($85,000) earn substantially less per year than family practitioners ($196,000) and general internists ($206,000), and that will help slow the growth of health-care spending if their roles increase compared with those of physicians.

Certified nurse-midwives also get a boost in the law that may lead more women to turn to them for a full range of primary-care services, not just reproductive care and deliveries.

At the moment, Medicare pays nurse-midwives 65 percent of what a physician is paid for a service, such as taking a Pap smear. Now, they will be reimbursed at 100 percent of the regular Medicare fee schedule.

Because most Medicare-covered women are beyond their reproductive years—younger disabled women, also Medicare beneficiaries, are the exception—few are cared for by nurse-midwives.

Those practitioners, however, fought for the change "as an equity issue," said Joanna King, director of government relations for the American College of Nurse-Midwives.

Both Medicaid and private insurers often follow Medicare's lead on payment matters. Consequently, King expects that "we may pretty quickly see some other adjustments to our payments." Today, Medicaid programs in about half the states reimburse nurse-midwives the same amount as physicians for a given procedure, with the rest paying reduced rates down to a floor of 65 percent.

The law's ultimate result may be to lure more nurses into midwifery and provide an incentive for them to establish free-standing practices in which they offer a full range of primary care services (which some already do).

Community clinics

The law also provides a huge boost—$11 billion over five years—to "community health centers." The first of these federally supported primary-care clinics opened in 1965. There are now 1,250 of them, in all states, serving about 20 million mostly low-income people.

Community health centers are staffed by the full range of health-care professionals, and provide primary care, dental care, addiction counseling and some social work services. At least half the members of their governing boards must be patients. While many patients are covered by Medicaid, Medicare or private insurance, about 40 percent have no insurance and pay out of pocket on a sliding-fee scale. Federal grants help cover the cost of their care.

At least some of the people who will remain uninsured after the law takes effect (including illegal immigrants) are likely to receive their care at community health centers.

Better Coordination

One cause of sub-optimal treatment and wasted money is the lack of coordination among private practitioners in the fee-for-service world (which is most of American medicine). The scope of that problem was made clear in an astonishing study published in 2009.

On average, a Medicare patient sees seven doctors, most of them specialists, in four different practices each year. Researchers at the Center for Studying Health System Change, in Washington, looked at what that might mean to a primary-care doctor who has many Medicare patients. They examined the experiences of 2,284 physicians in Medicare's fee-for-service program. Each doctor treated an average of 264 Medicare patients. Using billing information, they determined that for every 100 of those people a doctor treated, he or she might need to contact 99 other physicians in 53 practices to piece together what was happening with all of them.

That nightmarish prospect may partly explain the appallingly high "readmission rate" for Medicare patients. A study published in 2009 found that 20 percent of Medicare beneficiaries discharged from the hospital were readmitted within 30 days. Half of them had not visited a doctor during that period, when they were often in shaky health and taking new or higher-dose medication.

This might change if all the practitioners were in the same organization, or at least in a defined "web," with seamless access to patient records and a shared financial interest in making things work efficiently.

A new Center for Medicare and Medicaid Innovation will provide incentives for doctors, other professionals, hospitals, clinics, imaging centers, diagnostic labs, etc., to band together into "accountable care organizations" that would have total responsibility for a person's health care. Medicare would pay them a single "bundled" fee per patient, and in turn they would share in any savings that might accrue to Medicare as a result of not paying for every clinic visit, test and procedure.

To gain such savings, accountable-care organizations would have to keep patients healthy and out of the hospital and emergency room. That, in turn, would require health-care workers to perform services generally not done by doctors (or done only occasionally), such as home visits, medication monitoring, dietary counseling and intensive patient education.

The iron laws of economics suggest that only large organizations (or contractual arrangements among smaller ones) will be able to offer this kind of soup-to-nuts care. At the moment, 46 percent of clinicians work in practices with one to three doctors. Just less than 20 percent are in practices with 11 or more doctors.

Lots of doctors are going to have to change their work arrangements before the "accountable care" model becomes the norm—if it ever does.

Better Information

The American Recovery and Reinvestment Act of 2009 provided incentives for doctors to use electronic health record (EHR) systems in their practices, and incentive payments already exist for practitioners who report quality-related measures to Medicare. The new law will penalize doctors who don't make such reports, starting in 2015.

The new law also calls for information to flow the other way, too.

Physicians participating in the now-voluntary Physician Quality Reporting Initiative will start receiving feedback reports about how their performance compares to others, and to guidelines, beginning in 2012.

There is also money for the creation and dissemination of "patient decision aids"—handouts, videos, computer programs, etc.—that will help patients understand their treatment options. That is part of the law's general intent to make medical care more "patient-centered."

In one of the more controversial parts of its quality agenda, the law establishes a Patient-Centered Outcomes Research Institute to underwrite and direct "comparative-effectiveness research" seeking to determine the best and most economical treatment for common diseases. While the law specifically says that comparative-effectiveness findings can't become mandates that tell doctors how to practice, many champions of reform think that such research is essential to improving care.

"Three key steps—wise standardization, meaningful measurement and respectful reporting—have transformed other industries, and we believe they can help health care as well," 12 of them wrote in the *New England Journal of Medicine* in January 2010.

Tort Reform

Many physicians think that "defensive medicine"—the tendency to overtest and overtreat out of fear of being sued—is a big driver of rising health-care costs and that tort reform should have been a central part of the new law. Other health policy experts disagree.

Regardless of who is right, the law gives a nod to the issue of medical malpractice. It does not set limits on jury awards in malpractice cases, as doctors have sought. But it provides $50 million for five-year demonstration grants to help states develop alternatives to tort litigation. However, the alternative—say, arbitration before a panel of medical experts, not a jury—can't be mandatory. The law stipulates that plaintiffs will be able to opt out and go to court—a condition that makes many experts think these demonstration projects won't amount to much.

— *David Brown*

CHAPTER 10

Preventive Measures: More Carrots and More Sticks

In addition to helping people obtain care when they get sick, the new law is intended to keep them healthier by expanding coverage of preventive services, supporting an array of public health initiatives, and giving individuals incentives to adopt better habits.

That means you could be screened for diseases such as breast and colon cancer without having to pay anything out of pocket. On the other hand, if you smoke, if you're obese, or if you do not control your cholesterol levels, your employer could increase your premiums. Meanwhile, if you're trying to diet, help is on the way: When you visit your favorite chain restaurant, the number of calories in each item will be listed on the menu.

Preventive Benefits

Beginning in 2010, health plans will be required to cover the entire cost of certain preventive services. The requirement does not immediately extend to employer-provided plans that were already in place when the law was enacted.

Which services will be covered? Part of that is left to the secretary of Health and Human Services, who must define the minimum benefits for insurance sold through an exchange. The secretary has a broad mandate to include preventive and wellness services and management of chronic conditions.

Other authorities also have a say, starting with the U.S. Preventive Services Task Force (USPSTF), a panel that was established to make recommendations based on scientific evidence. The new law says services rated "A" or "B" by the task force must be covered. An "A" rating indicates a "high certainty that the net benefit is substantial"; a "B" rating indicates "high certainty that the net benefit is moderate" or "moderate certainty that the net benefit is moderate to substantial." The recommendations vary based on an individual's characteristics, such as age and sex.

A tool that allows users to search the recommendations can be found on the task force's Web site at http://epss.ahrq.gov/PDA/index.jsp.

Here are some examples:

For a 50-year-old woman who uses tobacco and is sexually active, the recommendations include:

- Screening for cervical cancer
- Screening for colorectal cancer
- Screening for breast cancer with mammography
- Screening for Type 2 diabetes, if the patient has sustained blood pressure of greater than 135/80

For the same profile, services that do not meet that threshold:

- Screening for ovarian cancer
- Screening for bladder cancer
- Screening for pancreatic cancer in the absence of symptoms

For a 35-year-old man who does not smoke and is sexually active, the recommendations include:

- Screening for high blood pressure

POUND OF CURE?

The emphasis on preventive care is rooted in an old saying: An ounce of prevention is worth a pound of cure. By that logic, new spending on preventive efforts could save the nation a pile of money. And it seems obvious enough: Recognize the symptoms of heart disease and seek treatment before you suffer a heart attack, and you may be able to avoid huge hospital bills.

But it isn't that simple. The cost of screening everyone for a particular medical problem can exceed the savings associated with the relatively small number of people who actually have the problem. When tests come back positive, they often increase costs—at least in the short term—by prompting people to seek more tests or treatment they otherwise would have gone without.

"Although different types of preventive care have different effects on spending, the evidence suggests that for most preventive services, expanded utilization leads to higher, not lower, medical spending overall," wrote Douglas W. Elmendorf, director of the Congressional Budget Office, in 2009.

If preventive medicine increases life expectancy, the government could also end up losing money, because Americans would collect more Medicare and Social Security benefits.

Of course, preventive care is about more than saving money; it's also about helping people live longer, healthier lives.

- Screening for lipid disorders if the patient is at increased risk of coronary heart disease

For the same profile, services that do not meet that threshold:

- An electrocardiogram or treadmill test if the patient is at low risk for coronary heart disease
- Screening for testicular cancer
- Screening for prostate cancer

The new law will cover immunizations, as recommended by an advisory committee of the Centers for Disease Control and Prevention. It will cover preventive care for infants, children and adolescents, as recommended by another federal body, the Health Resources and Services Administration. For women, it would go beyond the recommendations of the U.S. Preventive Services Task Force to cover future recommendations of the Health Resources and Services Administration.

To Test or Not to Test?

Although covering medical screening may seem unambiguously good, it can be fraught with complications. Experts don't always agree on the evidence, scientific consensus can shift and politics can enter the picture. Tests carry risks as well as benefits, and it isn't always clear what to do with the results.

The discovery of the prostate-specific antigen 40 years ago, for example, paved the way for millions of men to receive PSA screenings for prostate cancer. Although it can't detect the actual disease, and only some prostate cancers are life-threatening, the test leads many men to undergo biopsies and traumatic surgeries.

In November 2009, the USPSTF ignited a controversy by issuing a new recommendation on mammograms: Women younger than 50 should no longer undergo the breast cancer screenings as a matter of routine, the task force said. The recommendation roiled the debate over the health-care bill, and some people said it raised the specter of government rationing. Lawmakers amended the legislation to protect women's access to mammograms and other preventive care, though the law is not quite as explicit as advertised.

The standards for minimum coverage for exchange-based insurance could become one of the next battlegrounds, giving commercial interests and patient advocacy groups fresh opportunities to try to shape coverage.

Medicaid and Medicare

The focus on preventive care extends to the government programs for the poor, elderly and disabled.

- Medicare will stop charging co-pays for preventative services. Federal incentives could lead Medicaid to do the same.
- Medicaid will help pregnant women quit smoking. The program will pay for counseling and tobacco-cessation drugs.
- Medicare beneficiaries will be entitled to annual wellness visits at which practitioners assess their health risks and map out personalized prevention agendas.
- Enrollees in Medicare Advantage plans—private plans that operate under contract to Medicare—could lose ancillary benefits such as free gym memberships. The government, which says it has overpaid Medicare Advantage plans, is cutting their reimbursements and wants the plans to give higher priority to other matters, such as reducing members' out-of-pocket expenses for core medical benefits.

Public Health Initiatives

The new law includes a variety of initiatives aimed at the population at large. They include research projects, a national education campaign focused on dental care, and grants for public health agencies to watch for outbreaks of infectious disease.

The most conspicuous may be the one that displays calorie counts on restaurant menus—along with the recommended daily caloric intake. The requirement will apply to chains with 20 or more locations, and the eateries will have to make other nutritional information available on request. Many vending machines will have to disclose calorie content, too.

Carrots and Sticks

The new law does not merely encourage Americans to shape up; it could put them under increasing pressure to do so. That could take the form of rewards and penalties amounting to thousands of dollars per family.

Although the law bans varying premiums based on individual health status, it contains a major exception.

Section 2705 begins blandly enough by condoning the type of workplace wellness programs that have become staples of many corporate human resources departments. Employers are free to help workers pay for gym memberships and smoking-cessation classes. They can reward employees for, say, taking diagnostic tests or receiving prenatal care.

But they also are permitted to dispense financial rewards based on "satisfaction of a standard related to a health status factor"—in other words, based on the results of health-related tests. Employees who pass the tests are rewarded, while employees who don't are not.

The reward can take myriad forms, including lower premiums and deductibles. One person's reward can be the flip side of another person's penalty—as the law puts it, "the absence of a surcharge."

A federal regulation promulgated during the administration of George W. Bush said employers could use such incentives, and the health-care overhaul gives it the blessing of explicit legislation. In addition, beginning in 2014, the new law increases the amounts allowed for rewards and penalties. Previously, they were limited to 20 percent of the premium, counting both the employer and employee contributions. Now, they can be as much as 30 percent. In addition, the secretaries of Health, Labor and the Treasury can jointly raise the ceiling to 50 percent.

- At 30 percent, a single employee whose annual premiums cost him and his employer the national average of $4,824 could have $1,447 riding on test results. The new law raises the stakes by $482. At 50 percent, the same employee could have $2,412 on the line.
- At 30 percent, a family with the average premium of $13,375 could have $4,012 at risk, up $1,338 as a result of the new law. At 50 percent, the same family could have $6,688 on the line.

How common are such programs? Only 3 or 4 percent of large employers have been giving employees incentives to meet targets for weight, blood pressure and cholesterol levels, but about one in seven is considering doing so, according to a survey released in March 2010 by benefits consultant Towers Watson and the National Business Group on Health, a coalition of big employers.

The provision was sought by large employers and insurers. For supporters, it was partly a matter of principle: Why should non-smokers be forced to subsidize smokers through insurance premiums? Why should people who eat broccoli subsidize people who eat Big Macs?

The provision was opposed by labor unions and groups devoted to combating serious illnesses, such as the American Heart Association and the American Cancer Society. They said employers could use the incentives to discriminate against workers who are at risk of problems such as heart disease, diabetes and stroke. They predicted that meeting fitness standards could be especially hard for single parents, people working two jobs, and residents of poor neighborhoods with less access to healthy foods. One way the tests could save employers money, critics said, is by motivating certain employees to quit their jobs or leave the employer's health plan.

The law requires employers to make special accommodations for people who have extenuating medical circumstances. The law also says the tests cannot be "a subterfuge for discriminating based on a health status factor." It isn't clear how regulators will determine whether incentives reward people for good behavior or punish them for bad genes.

Insurers serving the individual market will be permitted to use the same approach in a 10-state demonstration project. As early as 2017, government officials could give a green light to insurers in other states.

— *David S. Hilzenrath*

CHAPTER 11

In the Workplace: What It Means for Employers

Employers have stood at the center of the nation's health-care system for more than half a century—and it appears the new legislation will keep them in a major role for now, at least when it comes to paying the tab. About 60 percent of Americans under age 65 currently receive health insurance through the workplace, even though delivering coverage has become increasingly burdensome for employers. Businesses of all sizes have been strained by rising costs, while small businesses venturing into the insurance market face deeper hazards.

The new law promises big changes for small employers and smaller changes for large employers.

Access to an Exchange

Beginning in 2014, businesses with up to 100 employees will be able to buy coverage for them through new state-based marketplaces known as exchanges. Through 2015, states will be allowed to set the ceiling as low as 50 employees. Authors of the law hope insurers will compete to sell insurance in the exchanges, and that, collectively, small groups will gain the buying power of larger companies.

Once an employer is in an exchange, it can stay there even if it grows beyond 100 workers.

Health plans offered through the exchanges will have up to four levels of coverage—bronze, silver, gold and platinum. Employers can choose the level for employees, and individuals can then choose among plans offered at that level. (See Chapter 1.)

The employer will decide how much to contribute toward employee premiums.

Beginning in 2017, states will have the option of opening exchanges to employers with more than 100 workers. If granted access, businesses would have to decide how deeply involved they'd like to remain in the delivery of benefits. Do they want to be passive payers or active managers? If the exchanges function as intended, they could enable employers to offer workers a wider choice of plans. Over the long run, if big enough companies send employees to the exchanges, the shift could end up dismantling the employer-based model.

Tax Credits

Beginning in 2010, employers with as many as 25 employees and average wages of up to $50,000 will be able to obtain tax credits to help defray the cost of coverage. To qualify, the employer must pay at least 50 percent of the premiums.

The size of the credit will vary based on the number of workers in the company and their average annual pay. The maximum credit goes to employers with 10 or fewer employees and average annual pay of less than $25,000.

- Through 2013, the credit will be worth as much as 35 percent of the premiums paid by the employer, or as much as 25 percent in the case of tax-exempt groups.

WHAT'S IT GOT TO DO WITH EMPLOYERS?

Why do employers serve as a gateway to health care in the United States? It was no grand design that put them there, but rather a confluence of forces, including an accident of history.

The tradition has roots in the 19th century. If railroad, mining and lumber companies operating on remote frontiers hadn't provided care for their employees, the workers would have had no care, as Paul Starr recounts in *The Social Transformation of American Medicine*. In later eras, labor unions pressed industrial companies for benefits, while cries of socialism helped thwart proposed public options—much as they did in 2009.

During World War II, wage and price controls brought a watershed: They restrained businesses from raising cash compensation for workers but left a loophole for medical benefits. In the postwar era, Congress exempted employer-sponsored medical benefits from employees' income taxes. That ensured that job-based health care would become an American institution.

- Beginning in 2014, the credit will be worth as much as 50 percent of the premiums paid by the employer, or as much as 35 percent in the case of tax-exempt groups.

In 2014 and beyond, employers can receive the credits for only two years, and only if they cover workers through an exchange.

Penalties

Employers will not be required to provide health benefits, but employers that provide no coverage or skimpy coverage could incur a penalty.

It would be triggered if any employee ends up receiving a government subsidy to buy insurance through an exchange. (Employees can qualify for subsidies of their own if the employer's plan pays for less than 60 percent of covered medical expenses or if the premium the employer requires them to pay amounts to more than 9.5 percent or more of their income.)

The penalties will apply only to employers with at least 50 employees. They are divided into two scenarios:

- If the employer does not offer coverage, the penalty will be $2,000 times the number of full-time employees in the business, not counting the first 30.
- If the employer offers coverage, the penalty will be the lesser of: (a) $2,000 times the number of full-time employees excluding the first 30, or (b) $3,000 times the number of employees receiving subsidies in an exchange.

Employers might conclude that paying the penalties is cheaper than paying premiums, and it is not clear how much incentive the penalties will give employers to offer coverage. In 2009, employers' share of worker premiums averaged $4,045 for single coverage and $9,860 for family coverage, according to a survey by the Kaiser Family Foundation. But the fact is, employers have paid those premiums in the absence of penalties to make themselves more competitive in the labor market.

Vouchers

Employers offering marginally affordable coverage will be required to give certain employees vouchers to buy coverage in the exchange.

Those vouchers will be for employees who fall below 400 percent of the federal poverty level and who would be spending 8 to 9.8 percent of their income on premiums if they enrolled in the employer's health plan. The voucher will be worth the amount the employer ordinarily would have paid toward the employee's coverage.

If employees take the vouchers to the exchange and also qualify for government subsidies, the employer would not incur a penalty.

Dependents

Like health plans in the individual market, group health plans must cover enrollees' children up to age 26. This requirement might entail added costs for employers, but it might help them, too, by bringing younger, healthier people into their pools.

Retirees

Until 2014, the law gives employers financial incentives to cover retirees who are at least 55 years old but not yet old enough to qualify for Medicare. Employers can obtain federal reimbursement for some of the expenses they incur caring for early retirees and members of their families, including surviving spouses.

The offer is good while the money lasts: The government has set aside $5 billion for the program. Employers will have to use the reimbursements to reduce premiums, co-payments, deductibles or other health-plan costs. Until the government translates the provision into clearer regulatory language, it is hard to say precisely how the amount of individual reimbursements would be determined.

Meanwhile, employers will lose the ability to claim tax deductions on top of federal subsidies they receive for retirees' prescription drug coverage. The deductions could be viewed as a double-dip. Some companies have begun taking big write-offs to account for the change.

Waiting Periods

Beginning in 2014, employers will be prohibited from requiring new hires to wait more than 90 days before receiving health benefits.

Automatic Enrollment

Beginning in 2014, employers with more than 200 full-time employees must make sure that workers are not left out of their health plans inadvertently. If those employers offer coverage, they must automatically enroll workers. If workers don't like the coverage, they can opt out.

Wellness Incentives

Beginning in 2014, the law will allow employers to increase financial incentives for employees to meet wellness standards. The incentives, which could take the form of differences in premiums and deductibles, would reward employees for passing health-related tests and penalize them for failing the tests. The law does not specify what tests employers may use—within certain parameters, it leaves that to employers—but the targets might include such measures as weight, blood pressure, cholesterol and tobacco usage. (See Chapter 10 on prevention and wellness.)

Excise Tax

The law imposes an excise tax on the richest health plans, or Cadillac plans. The tax is intended to slow the growth of medical spending. The tax initially hits individual coverage with premiums of more than \$10,200 and family coverage with premiums of more than \$27,500. However, the tax is not scheduled to take effect until 2018. That gives Congress eight years to revisit the issue—and employers eight years to prepare. Will employers reduce the value of their benefit packages, as proponents of the tax hoped? If so, will they make it up to workers by raising cash compensation?

WHY SMALL EMPLOYERS PAY MORE FOR INSURANCE

When it comes to buying insurance, small employers have some of the same vulnerabilities as people in the individual market: Without bargaining power and unable to spread risk across large numbers of people, they can pay a relatively steep price for age or illness. One major medical problem in the group can jeopardize the affordability of coverage for all. When they don't want to renew small businesses' policies, insurers essentially make them an offer they can't accept—raising premiums to prohibitive levels.

The system might work for small businesses filled with young, healthy people, but youth and good health don't last forever. And while many states offer at least some protections for small businesses, the rules vary widely.

In 2009, fewer than half (46 percent) of businesses with three to nine workers offered health benefits, while almost all (95 percent) with 50 or more employees provided coverage, according to a survey by the Kaiser Family Foundation and the Health Research & Educational Trust.

Large employers command a much stronger position. Their numbers give them market clout, and they are better able to absorb the financial shock when members of the group suffer catastrophic illness. But even the largest employers have had trouble controlling costs. Medical expenses detract from profits and wages. Internationally, the cost of employee health benefits undermines American competitiveness.

Former Chrysler chairman Lee Iacocca put the issue in perspective years ago when he said that U.S. automakers spent more per car on health care than on steel.

A Break on the "Hidden Health Tax"

Employers have long paid what policy wonks commonly call a hidden health tax; as a result of the legislation, they stand to receive a hidden tax cut. The hidden tax is the amount they have been paying through inflated hospital charges and other fees to cover the cost of emergency and other care for the uninsured. The legislation is projected to reduce the number of uninsured, and that could translate into savings for those who have private insurance.

However, there could also be a counter-effect if the expansion of Medicaid prompts providers to increase charges for patients with private insurance.

Bending the Curve

The bill includes an array of provisions meant to make the health-care system more efficient—for example, research as to what works and what doesn't in the practice of medicine, known as comparative effectiveness. (See Chapter 8.) Whether the legislation saves big employers money will depend largely on the law's indirect or systemic effects as opposed to any provisions aimed narrowly at employers.

(See Chapter 4 for more about the law's impact on insurance premiums.)

Grandfathering

When he was campaigning to overhaul health care, President Obama often said that if you like your coverage, you can keep it. He was trying to neutralize fears about change, especially for those content with their employer-sponsored coverage.

As a general rule, health plans in existence when Obama signed the law are grandfathered, meaning they are not required to comply with new requirements. The general rule, however, is riddled with exceptions: Some new requirements will apply to grandfathered plans.

For example, over time the legislation prohibits all employer plans from using some of the simplest cost-saving devices: lifetime and annual limits on the dollar value of coverage.

In addition, the law leaves a basic question unanswered: What would cause a health plan, including an employer-sponsored plan, to lose its grandfathered status? Would it take something as big as, say, switching from Aetna to Cigna? Or switching from one Aetna plan to another? Or could it happen if an employer changed something as small as the co-payment for a specific brand-name drug?

Those questions are among many that will be left to the rule makers.

When health plans of small employers lose grandfathered status, they will have to meet the requirements of the essential health benefits package, the floor for coverage offered through the exchanges.

Because employers are likely to change their plans sooner or later—benefits seldom stay frozen for long—it is probably just a matter of time before many employer-based plans must conform to something approaching the full set of new rules.

— *David S. Hilzenrath*

CHAPTER 12

Medicaid's Expansion: The Impact on the States

Aware that numerous states face yawning budget gaps, many Americans are wondering what the new health-care law will mean for their home states—and their state taxes.

The State Divide

Driven by the overall rise in medical expenses, a recession-fueled increase in enrollments and people's growing reliance on the program to pay for nursing home care, Medicaid costs have been gobbling up an increasing share of state budgets. The new law's plan to expand the joint state-federal program looks at first glance as though it could exacerbate that problem.

But the law's impact is more nuanced than it is has been made out to be. States will pick up some of the costs of insuring more people through Medicaid, but their portion for covering them will be much smaller than their share of the Medicaid responsibility today. In fact, some say the government's move to shoulder more Medicaid costs may be a step toward eventual federalization of the program, a move that would relieve state taxpayers.

As it now stands, the government covers half the cost of Medicaid in the wealthiest 14 states, and increasingly larger shares in the other states, with the poorest paying only a quarter of the cost.

There is also a wide variation among the states when it comes to Medicaid eligibility. In Alabama, Florida, Georgia, Missouri, Texas and Virginia, among others, parents who earn more than a third of the poverty level—about $7,500 for a family of four—are ineligible for Medicaid, meaning that only disabled or truly indigent adults qualify. By contrast, Connecticut, Maine, Minnesota, New Jersey, New York and Wisconsin enroll parents up to at least 150 percent of the poverty level, or about $33,000 for a family of four.

A New National Standard

The new law brings the country up to a common threshold.

In 2014, everyone earning 133 percent of the poverty level or less will be eligible for Medicaid. In today's dollars, that translates to $29,300 for a family of four or $14,400 for a single adult. It is estimated that this will bring 16 million more people into Medicaid—about half the number who are expected to receive insurance under the new law.

The federal government will pick up the vast majority of the cost of the "newly eligible" people: 100 percent from 2014 to 2016; 95 percent in 2017; 94 percent in 2018; 93 percent in 2019; and 90 percent in 2020 and subsequent years. (The "Cornhusker Kickback," which would have given Nebraska special terms, was stripped out of the legislation.)

The government will, for the most part, continue paying states under their existing formulas for people who join the Medicaid rolls in 2014 but who would have been eligible under the states' old rules—people who come forward to sign up because of the requirement that everyone have insurance.

Meanwhile, the federal government will relieve the states of much of their responsibility when it comes to the Children's Health Insurance Program (CHIP). The government now pays 65 percent to 83 percent of the cost, depending on a state's wealth. But starting in 2015, the federal share will increase by 23 percentage points, relieving a dozen states of all costs. Over time, CHIP may dissolve entirely as working-class families seek coverage in the exchanges instead. (See Chapter 5 for more about the impact of the new law on coverage for children.)

The Quest for Fairness

The impact will vary greatly. States that have had narrow eligibility standards will be adding far more people to their rolls, and nearly all those people will count as newly eligible and will therefore qualify for the higher federal contribution, starting at 100 percent and dropping to 90 percent in 2020. Even the states' small portion of the cost for people who are newly eligible for Medicaid will be significant. For instance, experts estimate that if the law went into effect immediately, 1 million people would fall into that group in Texas; the state's eventual 10 percent share for them would be about $370 million per year. (Texas already spends about $6 billion per year on Medicaid.)

Seen from another standpoint, though, the states that have had stringent eligibility rules until now will do well: Under the new law, the federal government will be paying a far greater share than it does now to cover a large additional swath of their populations— and a greater share than it will pay in states that have had broader eligibility. In Texas, officials estimate that for every additional dollar the state will spend for expanded Medicaid, the federal government will spend $6—resulting in a surge of federal money into that state.

This makes for some inequities—a point that Republican Scott Brown capitalized on in his upset Senate victory in Massachusetts, noting the overhaul would be unfair to states such as his that have already done a lot to expand coverage. For instance, the federal government will be paying 100 percent, and later 90 percent, to cover parents living at the poverty level in Virginia, because the state's rules have been so stringent that such a family will be newly eligible. But in Minnesota, which already covers families who earn up to double the poverty level, the federal government will cover parents at the poverty level under its existing formula for that state: 50 percent.

This disparity will be exacerbated by the "woodwork effect": In states that have had broad eligibility, many people who qualified for Medicaid did not enroll, but will soon come out of the woodwork to sign up because of the new requirement to obtain insurance. Because these people are not newly eligible, their states will not receive the higher federal match.

The legislation's authors tried to mitigate this unfairness. For instance, states that have already expanded eligibility to the poverty level will receive a phased-in increase of the federal share for covering childless adults so that they will, by 2020, get the same 90 percent portion that other states will then be receiving. States that have been covering people above 133 percent of the poverty level also will save some money because, come 2014, they will be allowed to lower that to the new national threshold and instead let people above that level buy insurance in the new state-based exchanges.

Still, states that have had narrower eligibility until now will, overall, be receiving a disproportionately larger share of federal aid than they do under current formulas.

What About Other State Programs?

Several states, including Connecticut, Pennsylvania and Washington, have had programs that provide coverage to adults who are not eligible for state Medicaid. Most of these programs probably will dissolve with the arrival of the new law's main provisions in 2014, when people will either qualify for Medicaid, if their income is below 133 percent of the poverty level, or will be able to buy insurance in the exchanges with the help of subsidies.

The new law does give states the option of continuing to offer separate programs for people between 133 percent and 200 percent of the poverty level. This "basic health plan" will have to offer the same essential benefits required of plans in the exchanges and will not be allowed to charge people more in premiums than they would have paid in the exchanges. States would receive 95 percent of the federal money that otherwise would have gone toward subsidies for people in the basic plan. This option will probably hold little appeal for most states, because it would carry an extra cost for them. But it will be an option for states that decide that people in this income bracket are not well served by the exchanges.

The law also lets states opt out of the exchanges in favor of a different approach—but only if they can achieve near-universal coverage with the same minimum benefits that are offered in the exchanges, and without increasing the federal deficit.

Are Immigrants Eligible for Expanded Medicaid?

The rules will remain the same as today: Illegal immigrants are not eligible for Medicaid, although there is an exception for childbirth care. Legal immigrants must wait five years before becoming eligible.

Will Expanding Medicaid Overwhelm the System?

This is a real concern. As it is, many physicians decline to take Medicaid patients, saying the reimbursement rates are too low. To address this, the law raises Medicaid payment rates for primary care doctors to Medicare levels, for 2013 and 2014.

What About Long-Term Care?

The law makes it easier for states to use Medicaid money for home- or community-based care for the elderly and disabled instead of having to institutionalize them. (See Chapter 7.) This could relieve the surge in Medicaid's nursing-home costs, though more people may also seek home-based Medicaid care once they realize it is covered.

What Else Might Go Wrong?

As much as the law attempts to limit the impact on state budgets, it is possible that the costs will outpace predictions, if the insurance mandate leads even more people than expected to sign up. There will also be administrative headaches as states try to determine whether someone is newly eligible or would have qualified under the old rules.

"States are shrugging and saying, 'We just don't know how it's going to work,' " said Scott D. Pattison, executive director of the National Association of State Budget Officers. "It's a real concern, about being able to analyze what their future costs will be."

— Alec MacGillis

CHAPTER 13

Paying for It:
Taxes, Penalties and Spending Cuts

According to official estimates, the new health-care law will spend $938 billion over the next decade to extend health insurance to millions of people who currently lack access to affordable coverage through employers. A little more than half of the money will finance tax credits and other subsidies to help small businesses and consumers buy insurance, primarily through new state-run marketplaces, or exchanges. The rest of it will pay for more people to obtain government coverage through Medicaid and other health programs for the poor and elderly.

The insurance expansion will be financed through a multitude of provisions that either reduce spending on existing government programs—primarily Medicare—or impose new taxes and penalties on individuals and businesses. Together, those provisions will generate more than $1 trillion over the next decade, slightly more than the total cost of the new programs. Any leftover cash will go toward reducing the enormous deficits projected for the rest of the federal budget during that period.

New Taxes and Penalties

Targeting high earners:

For the most part, lawmakers sought to pay for the reforms by siphoning money out of existing government health-care expenditures. The one big exception is the imposition of new taxes on adjusted gross incomes over $200,000 a year for individuals and $250,000 for families. These high earners—who make up less than 2 percent of all taxpayers—will be hit with two new taxes:

Higher Medicare payroll tax. Starting in 2013, the existing 1.45 percent tax for Medicare hospitalization insurance will increase to 2.35 percent on earnings over the thresholds set in the law. So an individual making $250,000 a year would pay 1.45 percent on the first $200,000 and 2.35 percent on the remaining $50,000. Similarly, a couple earning $300,000 a year would pay 1.45 percent on the first $250,000 and 2.35 percent on the remaining $50,000.

New Medicare tax on investment income. Also starting in 2013, high earners will have to pay a 3.8 percent Medicare "contribution" on unearned income, including interest, dividends, annuities, royalties, rents and capital gains. The tax will be owed on whichever is less: net investment income or modified adjusted gross income over the threshold. For individuals, the threshold is $200,000; for joint filers, it is $250,000. This tax adds a third threshold, of $125,000, for married individuals filing separate returns.

Because the income thresholds will not rise with inflation, the percentage of taxpayers subject to both of the new levies will grow over time.

Reducing existing tax breaks for health care:

The government currently uses the tax code to subsidize health

A LAW THAT'S PAID FOR?

By 2019, when the new law is fully implemented, the coverage expansion will cost about $215 billion a year. The savings and new revenue, meanwhile, will add up to about $230 billion a year. Because the financing stream is projected to grow faster than the cost of the new programs, the Congressional Budget Office says the Patient Protection and Affordable Care Act is fully paid for, both now and in the foreseeable future, and that it is not likely to worsen the government's gloomy budget picture. However, cost estimates for such complicated and sprawling legislation are highly uncertain, and policy experts disagree about their reliability.

insurance and medical care. Several provisions in the law will reduce those benefits:

New tax on expensive employer-provided health insurance, or "Cadillac" plans. The tax-free treatment of employer-based coverage is the single largest loophole in the tax code, exempting benefits that would generate more than $200 billion a year in revenue if taxed as income. If you are insured through work, you may not even know how much your employer spends on your policy.

That will change in 2011, when employers will have to report the cash value of health benefits on a worker's W-2 form. And, starting in 2018, insurance policies that cost more than $10,200 for individual coverage and $27,500 for family coverage—far more than the national average—will be subject to a 40 percent excise tax on the portion of the premiums that exceed that threshold.

The tax will be imposed on insurers who sell those policies and they are likely to pass on the added cost to consumers. Therefore, economists believe employers and their workers will choose less expensive health plans and shift the leftover cash to wages. Congressional tax analysts think most of the revenue from this provision will come from people paying income taxes on higher wages.

Many economists say this provision will help reduce overall spending on health care by steering people away from Cadillac plans that encourage overuse of medical services because they cover every office visit and procedure.

Changes to health savings accounts (HSAs) and other employer-sponsored medical savings arrangements. Starting in 2011, these accounts will no longer be used to pay for over-the-counter drugs, even those prescribed by a physician. In addition, penalties on non-allowable disbursements from such accounts will be taxed at 20 percent instead of 10 percent. And starting in 2013, workers who receive money from their employers to supplement health care and other benefits, known as flexible spending arrangements, will no longer be able to receive unlimited sums tax-free. Instead, these FSAs will be limited to $2,500 a year.

Higher threshold for deducting medical expenses. Currently, taxpayers must spend at least $7\frac{1}{2}$ percent of their annual income on medical expenses before they can claim a deduction from their income taxes. Starting in 2013, that threshold will increase to 10 percent of adjusted gross income for people younger than 65. In 2017, the threshold will rise for senior citizens as well.

Paying for new coverage mandates:

The goal of the health-care law is to extend insurance coverage to virtually every American citizen. Several new fees are designed to reinforce that goal or to extract contributions from industries that will profit from it.

New penalty for not obtaining insurance. By 2016, individuals who cannot provide proof of insurance will face penalties of $695 a year or $2\frac{1}{2}$ percent of income, whichever is greater. Families will face an annual maximum of $2,085 or $2\frac{1}{2}$ percent of income. (See Chapter 2.)

Paying for It

Expanding health coverage to millions of Americans will cost nearly $1 trillion over a decade. The government anticipates covering those costs through a combination of spending cuts, tax increases and penalties.

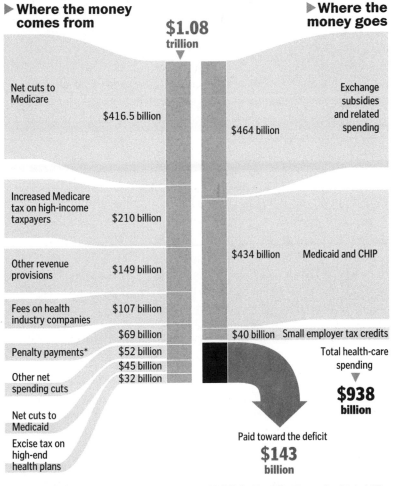

▶**Where the money comes from**

$1.08 trillion

▶**Where the money goes**

Net cuts to Medicare
$416.5 billion

Exchange subsidies and related spending
$464 billion

Increased Medicare tax on high-income taxpayers
$210 billion

Other revenue provisions
$149 billion

$434 billion   Medicaid and CHIP

Fees on health industry companies
$107 billion

$69 billion

$40 billion   Small employer tax credits

Penalty payments*
$52 billion

Total health-care spending

$45 billion

Other net spending cuts
$32 billion

$938 billion

Net cuts to Medicaid

Paid toward the deficit

Excise tax on high-end health plans

$143 billion

*From employers and individuals

SOURCE: Tax Foundation, Congressional Budget Office

WILL HEALTH-CARE REFORM REDUCE BUDGET DEFICITS?

Listening to President Obama and other Democrats, one might get the idea that health-care reform will generate such prodigious savings that the nation will soon be able to pay off its mounting foreign debt. On the other hand, just about any Republican will tell you that the new law is a budget-buster that will force future taxpayers to foot the bill for a vast new entitlement program.

The truth, as far as it is knowable, lies somewhere in between.

Two nonpartisan agencies—the Congressional Budget Office and the Joint Committee on Taxation—are the official scorekeepers for legislation that affects the federal budget. Using sophisticated computer models, the agencies have done their best to project the budgetary impact of the Patient Protection and Affordable Care Act.

Their conclusion, which is generally accepted by outside analysts, is that the law will increase overall government spending on health care in the first decade, but that it will slowly reduce that commitment thereafter, compared with the status quo, saving money in the long run.

How much money? Nearly $1.5 trillion over the next 20 years, Democrats say, using the CBO analysis.

But that turns out to be a lot less than it seems. The United States currently owes more than $8 trillion to China and other creditors. The CBO projects that the nation's debt will more than double over the next decade, exceeding $20 trillion by 2020. In a customary understatement, the agency has noted that savings from the health-care law are likely to erase only "a small share" of that problem.

There are other caveats. The CBO says the law puts "into effect a number of policies that might be difficult to sustain over a long period of time," particularly the reductions in Medicare spending. The legislation holds payments to many Medicare providers below the rate of inflation, then expects a new Independent Payment Advisory Board to cut even deeper without affecting services for seniors.

The law also does nothing to correct an existing formula that calls for payments to doctors who see Medicare patients to be cut by 21 percent in 2010. Lawmakers intend to fix that, at a cost of $200 billion over the next decade—a move that would wipe out all the short-term savings from the new legislation.

Health policy experts think the law contains many innovations that promise significant additional savings, far beyond CBO projections. Those savings could multiply if efficiencies in Medicare influence practices in the broader health-care system. Plus, no one really knows how prices will be affected by a changed landscape in which virtually everyone has insurance. Even a small downward shift in the rate of health-care inflation could dramatically improve the nation's budget outlook.

But at a time when the country is sinking rapidly into debt, many fiscal experts are worried. Lawmakers have voted to raise taxes and cut Medicare not to balance the budget, but to finance the biggest expansion of the social safety net in nearly half a century. That may eventually prove to be a wise investment, and the legislation's framers have tried to ensure that their reforms will not make the budget problem worse.

In the meantime, though, the red ink is still rising.

New penalty for not providing insurance. Starting in 2014, all but the smallest companies will face annual fees of $2,000 per worker if any of their employees qualify for federal health insurance subsidies. (See Chapter 11.)

New industry fees. In return for the opportunity to serve millions of new customers, certain players in the health-care industry have agreed to help finance reform. From 2011 to 2019, manufacturers and importers of brand-name drugs will pay annual fees totaling $27 billion. Starting in 2013, makers and importers of medical devices will pay a 2.3 percent excise tax on certain products. And from 2014 to 2019, insurance companies will pay annual fees totaling $60 billion.

In addition, starting in 2013, insurers that pay any of their executives annual salaries of more than $500,000 will owe additional taxes.

Other taxes

The law includes a number of small corporate tax increases unrelated to health-care reform. And while lawmakers for the most part rejected proposals to use the tax code to discourage unhealthy behavior, one such levy did make the final cut: Beginning July 1, 2010, customers of tanning salons will have to pay a 10 percent tax on those services.

Spending Reductions

In 2010 alone, the government expects to spend more than $500 billion on Medicare, the federal health-care program for people older than 65. The program ranks third in overall federal spending, behind Social Security and the Pentagon, and its cost is soaring as the U.S. population ages and overall medical costs rise. The law seeks to reduce Medicare spending in several ways.

Medicare Advantage

Intended to be a cost-saving alternative to traditional Medicare, Medicare Advantage is funded by the government but administered by private insurance companies. Over time, the program has proved to be significantly more costly than traditional Medicare; the health-care law will eliminate these excess payments. The approximately 11 million people who subscribe to Medicare Advantage plans could lose popular benefits such as gym memberships, but the changes will save the government nearly $140 billion over the next decade.

Payments to hospitals and other institutional providers

Anticipating millions of newly insured customers, hospitals

and other institutions have agreed to accept smaller increases in their Medicare payment rates over the next decade, saving the government nearly $200 billion. Billions more will be saved by cutting Medicare (and Medicaid) payments to hospitals that serve uninsured patients, whose numbers are expected to dwindle after 2014 when the law will require almost everyone to obtain insurance.

Independent payment advisory board

Dozens of other provisions aim to cut waste and encourage efficient delivery of services under Medicare. Lawmakers hope that such changes will further reduce costs, although the ideas are largely untested and congressional budget analysts have been reluctant to forecast significant savings. As a backstop, the law establishes an independent board with the authority to cut payments to Medicare providers even further if the program does not meet specified spending targets.

Other Funding Sources

The CLASS Act

Starting in 2012, the law will establish an insurance program for long-term care that is funded entirely by subscriber premiums. New subscribers will receive no benefits for at least five years, allowing the program to accumulate a large pool of cash, expected to total $70 billion by 2019.

Although this money is intended solely to pay benefits under the new insurance program (known as the Community Living Assistance Services and Supports Act), it is included in official estimates of the health-care law. So when budget analysts say the reform package will save the government $143 billion over the next decade, about half of that money is actually reserved for future CLASS Act benefits.

Student loan reforms

In the final weeks of the health-care debate, lawmakers tacked onto the legislation a series of changes to the federal student loan program. Of the $143 billion in promised savings from health-care reform, about $17 billion will come from the student loan provisions.

— *Lori Montgomery*

CHAPTER 14

The Abortion Fight: What the Compromise Means

The new health-care legislation was almost derailed in the final days before passage by disputes over whether it would provide federal funding for abortion. In the closing hours, the White House intervened with an executive order that brought on board enough lawmakers who oppose abortion to get the bill through. But there is lingering disagreement over the issue, with groups on each side deeply unhappy about the language.

The Problem

Under the Hyde Amendment, which took effect in 1977, federal funding cannot be used to pay for abortions, with an exception later added for cases of rape, incest or where the mother's life is in danger. The amendment prevents abortion from being covered by insurance plans for federal employees, by the Tricare plans for military families and by Medicaid. About a third of states do cover abortion for Medicaid enrollees, using separate state money.

The insurance system created by the new law does not lend itself to the same straightforward segregation of federal money. In the new state-based exchanges, people without employer-based coverage will be able to buy insurance using a combination of their own money and federal subsidies that most of them will receive.

Groups opposed to abortion initially expressed optimism that a larger government role in providing health insurance would mean greater sway for the Hyde Amendment. "When you expand the reach of federal funds, you expand the reach of federal policies" on abortion, said Richard Doerflinger of the U.S. Conference of Catholic Bishops.

The legislation's authors in the House initially sought to allow abortion coverage in the exchanges but require insurance companies to keep the federal subsidies separate from individual premiums. House members who oppose abortion dismissed that as an accounting gimmick and instead called for, and passed, an amendment by Rep. Bart Stupak (D-Mich.) that forbade any plans in the exchanges from covering abortion if they enrolled customers who received subsidies. Because the vast majority of people using the exchanges will qualify for subsidies, that would effectively keep any of those plans from including abortion insurance. Women could still buy separate abortion "riders," Stupak said, but abortion rights supporters doubted that companies would offer them and said that it was offensive to expect women to buy a separate rider in anticipation of having an abortion.

The Solution

With abortion rights groups adamantly opposed to the House language, the bill's authors in the Senate tried to bridge the gap, devising the language that ended up in the new law: Insurers can include abortion coverage in plans offered in the exchanges. But everyone who buys a plan that includes abortion insurance—whether a woman or man, of any age—will have to make two separate premium payments: one covering the bulk of the policy and another far smaller one, as little as $1 per month, for abortion coverage. The thinking is that this will further help insurers keep private premiums and federal money separate. (The law does not apply to employer-based insurance plans outside the exchanges, many of which cover abortion.) States will be allowed to prohibit abortion insurance in their exchanges (several states now bar such coverage in individual plans). And at least one of the two nationwide insurance plans to be offered through the exchanges will not include abortion coverage.

Both sides remain dissatisfied. Abortion-rights supporters predict that the law will effectively keep abortion coverage from being included in the exchanges, because insurers will find the two-payment rule cumbersome and consumers will consider the requirement bizarre or objectionable. "There will not be abortion coverage in the exchanges. There just won't be," said Linda J. Blumberg, a health policy analyst at the Urban Institute. The prospect of having no coverage for the procedure in the exchanges particularly concerns abortion-rights groups, given that the law envisions that more and more people will move into them over time. Women who now have abortion coverage, whether through their employers or in the individual market, could lose it if they shift to an exchange.

Antiabortion groups are also upset, saying that the two-payment rule is just another gimmick and that the government will for the first time be providing direct subsidies to help people buy plans that include abortion coverage. The groups are also unhappy about other provisions, including what they consider insufficient protection of health-care workers who do not want to take part in abortions and a loophole that they say could allow abortions in federally funded community health clinics, which have until now been forbidden to perform them.

To win over antiabortion House members, President Obama signed an executive order that instructs his administration to confirm that federal money in the exchanges is being kept separate from the premiums for abortion coverage; reaffirms laws that "prohibit discrimination against health-care facilities and health-care providers because of an unwillingness to provide, pay for, provide coverage of, or refer for abortions"; and forbids abortions at community health clinics. Antiabortion groups called the order an empty gesture.

What Will Happen?

Any number of outcomes are possible once the exchanges open for business in 2014. It could be that—as abortion-rights groups fear—few or no insurers will choose to include abortion coverage in their plans. In that case, women who buy insurance in the exchanges will have to pay for the procedure out of pocket. Today, a first-trimester abortion typically costs about $400. But the procedure can cost thousands of dollars in some cases, such as if a woman decides to terminate later in her pregnancy after learning of a major birth defect.

It is also possible, though, that some insurers will choose to offer plans with abortion coverage, particularly if the two-payment rule becomes a mere technical formality, unnoticed by consumers whose premiums are paid automatically.

Given the ongoing furor, it seems unlikely that the abortion issue will disappear by 2014. If insurers do offer plans that cover the procedure, abortion opponents will almost certainly do their best to publicize that fact: Plans in the exchanges that include the coverage could become a highly effective rallying point for the antiabortion movement.

—Alec MacGillis

CHAPTER 15

The Rest of the Story: Mental Health, Dental and More

Beyond the broad ways the law will change the health-care system, it is likely to have specific effects on certain realms of treatment and certain parts of the country. Among these are mental health services, dental services, pharmaceuticals, alternative and complementary medicine, and medical care in rural areas.

A brief tour of the impact on these areas hints at how far the law's tentacles reach into nearly all corners of the health-care system. In general, here are two ways of thinking about what lies ahead:

- The law's basic goal of improving access to health care for nearly all Americans will, for the most part, make it more available as well for people looking for services in these specific niches. (See Chapter 1 on expansion of coverage and Chapter 10 on preventive services.)
- Other provisions are aimed directly at one facet of health care or another. These are, for the most part, among the changes that different constituencies have prodded Congress to make for years. In some instances, separate legislation that lawmakers had previously introduced was folded into the law. Some industry lobbyists—and the constituencies they represent—are pleased with the end result. Others are less so.

Mental Health

More parity

The big deal for people who need mental health services is the significant strengthening of "parity"—that is, a level of insurance coverage equal to that for medical and surgical services. This builds on another law, which was enacted in 2008 and began taking effect in recent months. Under that legislation, insurance plans containing a mental health benefit were required to allow consumers the same number of visits as for other kinds of care—at no greater cost.

Mental health advocates hailed the law as a major improvement after a long era in which coverage of such treatment often had been skimpy, expensive or absent from health plans altogether. But advocates said it left two gaps. First, the parity requirement applied only to insurance provided through large employers. Second, and more significant, the law did not actually require insurers to provide mental health benefits, but only to provide the same level of coverage if they did.

The new law addresses both issues. It specifies that all health plans sold through the new state-based insurance exchanges must contain mental health services. That is likely to solve the first issue, because, starting in 2014, that is where most individuals and small businesses are expected to buy coverage. In addition, the law says that treatment for mental health problems and substance abuse must be included within a set of "essential health services," to be defined by the federal government, that every plan in an exchange will be required to cover.

More help within Medicaid

Until now, states have had the choice whether to include many mental health and substance abuse services within Medicaid. That will change in 2014, when the government will start requiring

Medicaid programs to cover both. It is not clear how generous that coverage will be, but it must be equivalent to whatever will be available in the exchanges. These benefits will apply to people who will be eligible to join Medicaid for the first time. Federal health officials will have to decide whether to give the same benefits to everyone else in the Medicaid program.

Another change in Medicaid probably will be particularly helpful to people severely impaired by a mental illness, according to mental health experts. Some of those people do not function well enough to earn much money, but they have not been able to join Medicaid in most of the country unless they had a child or qualified as disabled under Social Security rules—a slow and uncertain route. Under the new law, every state will be required by 2014 to enroll adults without dependent children, as long as their incomes are not too high.

Integrating mind and body

On a smaller scale, the law will set in motion several efforts, some of them experimental, to weave together mental health services with primary care. The basic idea is to keep tabs on all the treatment and medication used by people who have at least two chronic conditions. A serious, long-lasting mental illness qualifies as such a condition. This coordination is supposed to occur by creating interdisciplinary treatment teams or assigning patients to a "medical home"—that is, a site that will oversee the many facets of their care. The government will provide grants to try such approaches for patients covered by private insurance and Medicare. And states will be able to use the approaches, if they choose, under Medicaid.

Supporting research

The law will create a National Center of Excellence for Depression to sponsor research into the effectiveness of approaches for treating depression and bipolar disorder.

Dental Health

A few days before Congress took its final votes on the legislation, the president of the American Dental Association dispatched a letter to House Speaker Nancy Pelosi saying that the group opposed it. The bill was missing "a commitment to improve the oral health for those citizens at the lowest end of the economic ladder," the letter said.

For years, the group had urged the government to require states to provide dental coverage for adults under Medicaid. Americans who are poor tend to receive far less dental care than others. Just nine states included full dental benefits in 2009 for adults in Medicaid on an optional basis, while most offered coverage on a limited basis only in emergencies, and eight provided none at all.

In the end, the law does not require Medicaid to add such a benefit. In fact, advocates for dentists worry that some states that now include dental services for adults could drop them in the future, once the government starts requiring states to shoulder a fraction of the expense of extending Medicaid to many more people.

Instead, the law requires Medicaid programs to provide dental coverage to children, as they have in the past. It also will, starting in 2014, require any health plan sold through the state insurance exchanges to include "pediatric oral care," but none for adults. It remains unclear how much dental care will be covered for children and at what cost. That is one of many decisions the Health and Human Services Department must make when it defines the "essential health benefits."

A few other provisions of the law also will affect oral health. They include relatively small amounts of money to train more dentists and increase the faculty at dental schools. And from 2010 to 2104, the law will give the Centers for Disease Control and Prevention money to help states promote community-based oral health initiatives, such as adding fluoride to drinking water in places that lack it and providing sealants against tooth decay to schoolchildren.

Pharmaceuticals

Drug pricing

The major news relating to drug prices is what did not happen. The law does not contain either of two big ideas that some liberals have promoted for years as ways to lower prescription drug costs.

One of those absent ideas is "reimportation"—a circuitous path, forbidden by the government, through which pharmaceuticals are manufactured in the United States, then shipped to Canada or perhaps other countries that control drug prices. As a final step, they are sold back into the United States at lower prices than if they had been sold here in the first place.

Nor does the law hand the government a bigger role in setting drug prices for older Americans covered by Medicare. The House had wanted to assign the Health and Human Services Department to wield its bulk-purchasing power to negotiate directly with pharmaceutical companies for the drugs consumed as part of Medicare's Part D drug benefit. Instead, each private drug plan that has a contract with Medicare will continue to negotiate whatever prices it can with drugmakers.

Still, the law will impose financially on the pharmaceutical industry. Drug manufacturers will be required to chip in perhaps $105 billion over the first decade to help defray the cost of several aspects of the legislation, according to Avalere Health, a Washington-based consulting firm. Some health policy analysts predict that manufacturers could make up the difference by charging consumers higher prices.

New on the market

Other parts of the law will affect how quickly new drugs and biologics come onto the market. A biologic is a product—such as some injectable therapies for cancer, anemia or multiple sclerosis—that is synthesized from living organisms. For a new biologic, the law says that, starting right away, the Food and Drug Administration must give exclusive rights to data for 12 years to the company that manufactured it, before generic versions will be allowed.

After the patent term has elapsed, the FDA will have to rule quickly on applications from other manufacturers to copy the original—a change that, if successful, could more swiftly lower the price of biologics for consumers.

Alternative and Complementary Medicine

Health insurers have tended not to cover much alternative or complementary medicine—also known as integrative or natural medicine. The law will make a few changes—some helpful, others not—that will affect consumers of approaches such as acupuncture, massage therapy or vitamin regimens.

Practitioners such as chiropractors and acupuncturists have long complained that insurance often does not cover their services, even when it covers doctors who do the same thing. Under the new law, if an insurer contracts with such practitioners, it will have to cover any service that their professional license entitles them to provide. This requirement, effective in 2014, will apply only to new insurance policies. The law does not require insurers to include these practitioners in the first place.

On the other hand, the law could make it harder for some people to afford such services. Because insurance seldom covers what they want, some of the most enthusiastic proponents of alternative health therapies tend to buy bare-bones, catastrophic insurance policies—or none at all—and rely on flexible-spending accounts through their employers to pay for care on a pre-tax basis. The law will restrict how much money people can contribute to these accounts—$2,500, as of 2013, with the amount to grow over the years to account for inflation. In the meantime, the insurance mandate will require these consumers to buy more expensive coverage than they may want.

Rural Health

Americans who live in remote, rural communities are more prone than those elsewhere to be uninsured. Even if they have coverage, they tend to have less access to health care nearby. This is partly because fewer medical professionals live and work in such places. Experts have long disagreed about how much sophisticated treatment should be available in sparsely populated areas, and how far rural residents should be expected to travel if they need highly specialized care. A related debate has simmered for years over whether the Medicare and Medicaid programs pay enough to hospitals, doctors and other health-care workers in rural areas. The new law deals with many, if not all, of these questions.

The rural workforce

The law will, over half a dozen years starting in 2010, significantly increase funding to the longstanding National Health Service Corps, which forgives student loans for some doctors and dentists if they take jobs for a few years in parts of the country where health professionals are scarce. Another provision will provide $4 million per year in grants, from 2010 to 2013, to encourage medical schools to recruit students from rural areas—in hopes that they eventually will return home to work.

In addition, the law will, starting in 2011, alter several important rules for graduate medical education subsidies, provided through Medicare, that help pay to train medical residents. For the first time, for instance, some of these subsidies will be given as grants to place residents in community settings, including Rural Health Clinics.

The law also creates a National Health Care Workforce Commission, which will, among other things, study how to even out the distribution of health professionals among rural communities, cities and suburbs.

Higher pay

To coax more primary-care doctors into rural areas—and keep the ones who already are there—the Medicare program will pay 10 percent bonuses from 2011 to 2015 to those who work where physicians are scarce. (The bonuses also will go to primary-care physicians in city neighborhoods that are short on doctors.) And in 2010 and 2011, the government will give a total of $400 million extra to rural and other hospitals where Medicare's ordinary payment rates are low. Meanwhile, some rural doctors will be paid more because of a tweak in 2010 to one of the formulas that Medicare uses to determine its rates for physicians.

One more thing: The law tells a commission that advises Congress on Medicare policy to study whether the program is paying enough for services in rural areas.

— Amy Goldstein

CONCLUSION

Judging Success

As interminable as the health-care debate seemed through 2009 and in early 2010, the journey to a new system has only just begun.

The legislation reached the finish line only after a string of concessions succeeded in defusing opposition—and those very points of compromise could one day reemerge as points of contention if it becomes apparent that the law does not do enough to fix a broken system.

More immediate is the challenge of carrying out what the legislation does call for. The law gets off to a relatively quiet start: Several rules go into effect in the months after signing, but the biggest provisions—the individual coverage mandate, the insurance exchanges, the subsidies—do not take hold until 2014. It probably seems to many as though nothing much is going on—as though all the uproar was for naught.

But amid the apparent stasis, countless shifts are underway. The health-care industry is hard at work anticipating the law's impact. Insurers are calculating how to position themselves for the new market that will unfold; doctors and hospitals are discussing whether to organize themselves into the more closely coordinated, salary-based provider networks that the law encourages.

Most crucially, federal officials are beginning the formidable task of translating the law's broad strokes into specific regulations. Just what are the "essential benefits" that the exchanges' plans will need to provide? How will regulators calculate insurers' "medical loss ratios"—the amount they pay to cover claims—to determine whether they are seeking excessive profits? What factors will go into the "value index" that assesses which hospitals are deemed efficient and deserving of higher Medicare payments? In one area after another, much of the law's impact will remain in the hands of federal health officials.

Just as critical will be the construction of the new system. States will need to set up the exchanges where, starting in 2014, small businesses and people without employer coverage will be able to buy insurance. For states that already have robust regulatory systems this may be relatively easy; for others, it will be a daunting undertaking and one that threatens to undermine the law's goals, given that many of the uninsured live in less-regulated states.

Will state officials band together with the insurance industry as successfully as they did in Massachusetts to promote the individual mandate and explain to people how they can sign up for coverage? That effort—so central to the law's success—will almost certainly be complicated by resistance to the mandate in many parts of the country. And states and medical providers will need to prepare for a massive influx into Medicaid: In Texas alone, about 1 million more people will be eligible.

Meanwhile, as government and the health-care industry are trying to implement the law, the rest of us may wonder: How will we even know whether this new system is working? We would be well-advised, for starters, to put little credence in the propagandists of either camp who will be seizing on any upward or downward tick in insurance premiums over the next year or two to declare the law a success or failure before its main provisions even take effect.

But what about after that? If the law is working, the vast majority of uninsured people will have signed up for coverage. Insurers will increasingly resemble well-regulated public utilities, with a guaranteed base of customers coupled with new constraints on their rates and profits. They will be making enough money to stay in business, but may also employ fewer people to do the work that will be rendered largely irrelevant by the law: deciding whom to insure and whom not to.

And, if the law plays out the way many of its supporters envision, the exchanges will become over time the new foundation for health insurance, making obsolete the employer-based benefit system that has been dominant for decades. Larger companies will start buying their coverage in the exchanges, giving workers more standardized benefits and more choices. Over the even longer term, the whole expectation that employers provide health benefits may dissipate as more workers buy their own insurance in the exchanges and as employers make up in higher wages the savings they gain from no longer paying for health benefits.

If the law is not working so well, many Americans may begin skirting the mandate, either paying the noncompliance penalty or simply ignoring the requirement and waiting to see whether the government fines them. People who are inclined to buy insurance in the exchanges may find the premiums unaffordable, even with the subsidies. This will be especially true if healthier people decide not to buy coverage, leaving the exchanges to serve people who are sicker and more expensive to insure. Better-off people may decide to buy plans outside the exchanges, leaving the new system to become the domain of the less healthy and the working class—a safety net propped up by taxpayer subsidies, not the thriving marketplace envisioned by the law. If that happens, many insurers may avoid the exchanges, leaving few choices for consumers.

Already, many health-care experts fear the legislation may not work as intended—in particular, that it will not do enough to control costs, thereby leaving the rise in premiums unchecked and imperiling the whole effort to extend coverage. The law includes some cost-control measures, but, over and over again, lawmakers balanced their desire to slow medical spending against the political realities of getting their bills past a minefield of potential opposition from segments of the health-care industry.

Even though the exchanges will encourage more competition among insurers, the law does far less in taking on what many economists believe is the main dynamic driving costs higher: the market control exerted by medical providers and drug companies that charge far more for most procedures and products than their counterparts in other countries. To keep deep-pocketed pharmaceutical companies on its side, the Obama administration opted not to press for the right to negotiate drug prices in Medicare or to allow the re-importation of drugs from abroad at lower prices. And at the urging of hospitals and physicians, the administration did not push as hard as it could have for a government-run insurance plan, or "public option," that people could buy in the exchanges in addition to private plans. While supporters of the public option promoted it primarily as needed competition for private insurers, many economists think its biggest potential impact would have been its purchasing power in seeking lower rates from medical providers.

If costs continue to escalate, another confrontation may loom, this time with doctors, hospitals and drugmakers. That is occurring in Massachusetts, where the quest for near-universal coverage has succeeded, but costs have kept rising. As a result, the state is proposing new constraints on providers, from setting hospital rates to goading doctors to form networks in which they will be paid collectively to keep people healthy instead of charging for each treatment as they do in today's fragmented system.

This fight, and many others, may lie ahead. But first we will have to wait and see what comes of the Patient Protection and Affordable Care Act of 2010, the first comprehensive health-care overhaul in the history of the United States, and the nation's first attempt to provide coverage for nearly every citizen. For all its compromises and potential flaws, the law will change our country, starting now.

— *Alec MacGillis*

PART III

THE LAW

This summary was produced by the Congressional Research Service (CRS) of the Library of Congress after the Senate passed its health-care bill on Dec. 24, 2009. The House passed it on March 21, 2010.

* * *

H.R.3590

Title:
Patient Protection and Affordable Care Act

Sponsor:
Rep. Rangel, Charles B. [NY-15]
(introduced 9/17/2009) Co-sponsors (40)

Related Bills:
H.CON.RES.254, H.RES.1203,
H.R.3780, H.R.4872, S.1728

Latest Major Action:
Became Public Law No: 111-148

The Patient Protection and Affordable Care Act

Title I: Quality, Affordable Health Care for All Americans

Subtitle A: Immediate Improvements in Health Care Coverage for All Americans

(Sec. 1001, as modified by Sec. 10101) Amends the Public Health Service Act to prohibit a health plan from establishing lifetime limits or annual limits on the dollar value of benefits for any participant or beneficiary after January 1, 2014. Permits a restricted annual limit for plan years beginning prior to January 1, 2014. Declares that a health plan shall not be prevented from placing annual or lifetime per-beneficiary limits on covered benefits that are not essential health benefits to the extent that such limits are otherwise permitted.

Prohibits a health plan from rescinding coverage of an enrollee except in the case of fraud or intentional misrepresentation of material fact.

Requires health plans to provide coverage for, and to not impose any cost sharing requirements for: (1) specified preventive items or services; (2) recommended immunizations; and (3) recommended preventive care and screenings for women and children.

Requires a health plan that provides dependent coverage of children to make such coverage available for an unmarried, adult child until the child turns 26 years of age.

Requires the Secretary of Health and Human Services (HHS) to develop standards for health plans to provide an accurate summary of benefits and coverage explanation. Directs each health plan, prior to any enrollment restriction, to provide such a summary of benefits and coverage explanation to: (1) the applicant at the time of application; (2) an enrollee prior to the time of enrollment or re-enrollment; and (3) a policy or certificate holder at the time of issuance of the policy or delivery of the certificate.

Requires group health plans to comply with requirements relating to the prohibition against discrimination in favor of highly compensated individuals.

Requires the Secretary to develop reporting requirements for health plans on benefits or reimbursement structures that: (1) improve health outcomes; (2) prevent hospital readmissions; (3) improve patient safety and reduce medical errors; and (4) promote wellness and health.

Requires a health plan to: (1) submit to the Secretary a report concerning the ratio of the incurred loss (or incurred claims) plus the loss adjustment expense (or change in contract reserves) to earned premiums; and (2) provide an annual rebate to each enrollee if the ratio of the amount of premium revenue expended by the issuer on reimbursement for clinical services provided to enrollees and activities that improve health care quality to the total amount of premium revenue for the plan year is less than 85% for large group markets or 80% for small group or individual markets.

Requires each U.S. hospital to establish and make public a list of its standard charges for items and services.

Requires a health plan to implement an effective process for appeals of coverage determinations and claims.

Sets forth requirements for health plans related to: (1) designation of a primary care provider; (2) coverage of emergency services; and (3) elimination of referral requirements for obstetrical or gynecological care.

(Sec. 1002) Requires the Secretary to award grants to states for offices of health insurance consumer assistance or health insurance ombudsman programs.

(Sec. 1003, as modified by Sec. 10101) Requires the Secretary to establish a process for the annual review of unreasonable increases in premiums for health insurance coverage.

(Sec. 1004) Makes this subtitle effective for plan years beginning six months after enactment of this Act, with certain exceptions.

Subtitle B: Immediate Actions to Preserve and Expand Coverage

(Sec. 1101) Requires the Secretary to establish a temporary high risk health insurance pool program to provide health insurance coverage to eligible individuals with a preexisting condition. Terminates such coverage on January 1, 2014, and provides for a transition to an American Health Benefit Exchange (Exchange).

(Sec. 1102, as modified by Sec. 10102) Requires the Secretary to establish a temporary reinsurance program to provide reimbursement to participating employment-based plans for a portion of the cost of providing health insurance coverage to early retirees before January 1, 2014.

(Sec. 1103, as modified by Sec. 10102) Requires the Secretary to establish a mechanism, including an Internet website, through which a resident of, or small business in, any state may identify affordable health insurance coverage options in that state.

(Sec. 1104) Sets forth provisions governing electronic health care transactions. Establishes penalties for health plans failing to comply with requirements.

(Sec. 1105) Makes this subtitle effective on the date of enactment of this Act.

Subtitle C: Quality Health Insurance Coverage for All Americans

Part I: Health Insurance Market Reforms

(Sec. 1201, as modified by Sec. 10103) Amends the Public Health Service Act to prohibit preexisting condition exclusions. Prohibits discrimination on the basis of any health status-related factor. Allows premium rates to vary only by individual or family coverage, rating area, age, or tobacco use.

Requires health plans in a state to: (1) accept every employer and individual in the state that applies for coverage; and (2) renew or continue coverage at the option of the plan sponsor or the individual, as applicable.

Prohibits a health plan from establishing individual eligibility rules based on health status-related factors, including medical condition, claims experience, receipt of health care, medical history, genetic information, and evidence of insurability.

Sets forth provisions governing wellness programs under the health plan, including allowing cost variances for coverage for participation in such a program.

Prohibits a health plan from discriminating with respect to participation under the plan or coverage against any health care provider who is acting within the scope of that provider's license or certification under applicable state law.

Requires health plans that offer health insurance coverage in the individual or small group market to ensure that such coverage includes the essential health benefits package. Requires a group health plan to ensure that any annual cost-sharing imposed under the plan does not exceed specified limitations.

Prohibits a health plan from: (1) applying any waiting period for coverage that exceeds 90 days; or (2) discriminating against individual participation in clinical trials with respect to treatment of cancer or any other life-threatening disease or condition.

Part II: Other Provisions

(Sec. 1251, as modified by Sec. 10103) Provides that nothing in this Act shall be construed to require that an individual terminate coverage under a group health plan or health insurance coverage in which such individual was enrolled on the date of enactment of this Act.

Applies provisions related to uniform coverage documents and medical loss ratios to grandfathered health plans for plan years beginning after enactment of this Act.

(Sec. 1252) Requires uniform application of standards or requirements adopted by states to all health plans in each applicable insurance market.

(Sec. 1253, as added by Sec. 10103) Directs the Secretary of Labor to prepare an annual report on self-insured group health plans and self-insured employers.

(Sec. 1254, as added by Sec. 10103) Requires the HHS Secretary to conduct a study of the fully-insured and self-insured group health plan markets related to financial solvency and the effect of insurance market reforms.

(Sec. 1255, as modified by Sec. 10103) Sets forth effective dates for specified provisions of this subtitle.

Subtitle D: Available Coverage Choices for All Americans

Part I: Establishment of Qualified Health Plans

(Sec. 1301, as modified by Sec. 10104) Defines "qualified health plan" to require that such a plan provides essential health benefits and offers at least one plan in the silver level and at least one plan in the gold level in each Exchange through which such plan is offered.

(Sec. 1302, as modified by Sec. 10104) Requires the essential health benefits package to provide essential health benefits and limit cost-sharing. Directs the Secretary to: (1) define essential health benefits and include emergency services, hospitalization, maternity and newborn care, mental health and substance use disorder services, prescription drugs, preventive and wellness services and chronic disease management, and pediatric services, including oral and vision care; (2) ensure that the scope of the essential health benefits is equal to the scope of benefits provided under a typical employer plan; and (3) provide notice and an opportunity for public comment in defining the essential health benefits. Establishes: (1) an annual limit on cost-sharing beginning in 2014; and (2) a limitation on the deductible under a small group market health plan.

Sets forth levels of coverage for health plans defined by a certain percentage of the costs paid by the plan. Allows health plans in the individual market to offer catastrophic coverage for individuals under age 30, with certain limitations.

(Sec. 1303, as modified by Sec. 10104) Sets forth special rules for abortion coverage, including: (1) permitting states to elect to prohibit abortion coverage in qualified health plans offered through an Exchange in the state; (2) prohibiting federal funds from being used for abortion services; and (3) requiring separate accounts for payments for such services.

(Sec. 1304, as modified by Sec. 10104) Sets forth definitions for terms used in this title.

Part II: Consumer Choices and Insurance Competition Through Health Benefit Exchanges

(Sec. 1311, as modified by Sec. 10104) Requires states to establish an American Health Benefit Exchange that: (1) facilitates the purchase of qualified health plans; and (2) provides for the establishment of a Small Business Health Options Program (SHOP Exchange) that is designed to assist qualified small employers in facilitating the enrollment of their employees in qualified health plans offered in the small group market in the state.

Requires the Secretary to establish criteria for the certification of health plans as qualified health plans, including requirements for: (1) meeting market requirements; and (2) ensuring a sufficient choice of providers.

Sets forth the requirements for an Exchange, including that an Exchange: (1) must be a governmental agency or nonprofit entity that is established by a state; (2) may not make available any health plan that is not a qualified health plan; (3) must implement procedures for certification of health plans as qualified health plans; and (4) must require health plans seeking certification to submit a justification of any premium increase prior to implementation of such increase.

Permits states to require qualified health plans to offer additional benefits. Requires states to pay for the cost of such additional benefits.

Allows a state to establish one or more subsidiary Exchanges for geographically distinct areas of a certain size.

Applies mental health parity provisions to qualified health plans.

(Sec. 1312, as modified by Sec. 10104) Allows an employer to select a level of coverage to be made available to employees through an Exchange. Allows employees to choose to enroll in any qualified health plan that offers that level of coverage. Permits states to allow large employers to join an Exchange after 2017.

(Sec. 1313, as modified by Sec. 10104) Requires an Exchange to keep an accurate accounting of all activities, receipts, and expenditures and to submit to the Secretary, annually, a report concerning such accountings. Requires the Secretary to take certain action to reduce fraud and abuse in the administration of this title. Requires the Comptroller General to conduct an ongoing study of Exchange activities and the enrollees in qualified health plans offered through Exchanges.

Part III: State Flexibility Relating to Exchanges

(Sec. 1321) Requires the Secretary to issue regulations setting standards related to: (1) the establishment and operation of Exchanges; (2) the offering of qualified health plans through Exchanges; and (3) the establishment of the reinsurance and risk adjustment programs under part V.

Requires the Secretary to: (1) establish and operate an Exchange within a state if the state does not have one operational by January 1, 2014; and (2) presume that an Exchange operating in a state before January 1, 2010, that insures a specified percentage of its population meets the standards under this section.

(Sec. 1322, as modified by Sec. 10104) Requires the Secretary to establish the Consumer Operated and Oriented Plan (CO-OP) program to foster the creation of qualified nonprofit health insurance issuers to offer qualified health plans in the individual and small group markets. Requires the Secretary to provide for loans and grants to persons applying to become qualified nonprofit health insurance issuers. Sets forth provisions governing the establishment and operation of CO-OP program plans.

(Sec. 1324, as modified by Sec. 10104) Declares that health insurance coverage offered by a private health insurance issuer shall not be subject to federal or state laws if a qualified health plan offered under the CO-OP program is not subject to such law.

Part IV: State Flexibility to Establish Alternative Programs

(Sec. 1331, as modified by Sec. 10104) Requires the Secretary to establish a basic health program under which a state may enter into contracts to offer one or more standard health plans providing at least the essential health benefits to eligible individuals in lieu of offering such individuals coverage through an Exchange. Sets forth requirements for such a plan. Transfers funds that would have gone to the Exchange for such individuals to the state.

(Sec. 1332) Authorizes a state to apply to the Secretary for the waiver of specified requirements under this Act with respect to health insurance coverage within that state for plan years beginning on or after January 1, 2017. Directs the Secretary to provide for an alternative means by which the aggregate amounts of credits or reductions that would have been paid on behalf of participants in the Exchange will be paid to the state for purposes of implementing the state plan.

(Sec. 1333, as modified by Sec. 10104) Requires the Secretary to issue regulations for the creation of health care choice compacts under which two or more states may enter into an agreement that: (1) qualified health plans could be offered in the individual markets in all such states only subject to the laws and regulations of the state in which the plan was written or issued; and (2) the issuer of any qualified health plan to which the compact applies would continue to be subject to certain laws of the state in which the purchaser resides, would be required to be licensed in each state, and must clearly notify consumers that the policy may not be subject to all the laws and regulations of the state in which the purchaser resides. Sets forth provisions regarding the Secretary's approval of such compacts.

(Sec. 1334, as added by Sec. 10104) Requires the Director of the Office of Personnel Management (OPM) to: (1) enter into contracts with health insurance issuers to offer at least two multistate qualified health plans through each Exchange in each state to provide individual or group coverage; and (2) implement this subsection in a manner similar to the manner in which the Director implements the Federal Employees Health Benefits Program. Sets forth requirements for a multistate qualified health plan.

Part V: Reinsurance and Risk Adjustment

(Sec. 1341, as modified by Sec. 10104) Directs each state, not later than January 1, 2014, to establish one or more reinsurance entities to carry out the reinsurance program under this section. Requires the Secretary to establish standards to enable states to establish and maintain a reinsurance program under which: (1) health insurance issuers and third party administrators on behalf of group health plans are required to make payments to an applicable reinsurance entity for specified plan years; and (2) the applicable reinsurance entity uses amounts collected to make reinsurance payments to health insurance issuers that cover high-risk individuals in the individual market. Directs the state to eliminate or modify any state high-risk pool to the extent necessary to carry out the reinsurance program established under this section.

(Sec. 1342) Requires the Secretary to establish and administer a program of risk corridors for calendar years 2014, 2015, and 2016 under which a qualified health plan offered in the individual or small group market shall participate in a payment adjusted system based on the ratio of the allowable costs of the plan to the plan's aggregate premiums. Directs the Secretary to make payments when a plan's allowable costs exceed the target amount by a certain percentage and directs a plan to make payments to the Secretary when its allowable costs are less than target amount by a certain percentage.

(Sec. 1343) Requires each state to assess a charge on health plans and health insurance issuers if the actuarial risk of the enrollees of such plans or coverage for a year is less than the average actuarial risk of all enrollees in all plans or coverage in the state for the year. Requires each state to provide a payment to health plans and health insurance issuers if the actuarial risk of the enrollees of such plan or coverage for a year is greater than the average actuarial risk of all enrollees in all plans and coverage in the state for the year. Excludes self-insured group health plans from this section.

Subtitle E: Affordable Coverage Choices for All Americans

Part I: Premium Tax Credits and Cost-Sharing Reductions

Subpart A: Premium Tax Credits and Cost-Sharing Reductions
(Sec. 1401, as modified by section 10105) Amends the Internal Revenue Code to allow individual taxpayers whose household income equals or exceeds 100%, but does not exceed 400%, of the federal poverty line (as determined in the Social Security Act [SSA]) a refundable tax credit for a percentage of the cost of premiums for coverage under a qualified health plan. Sets forth formulae and rules for the calculation of credit amounts based upon taxpayer household income as a percentage of the poverty line.

Directs the Comptroller General, not later than five years after enactment of this Act, to conduct a study and report to specified congressional committees on the affordability of health insurance coverage.

(Sec. 1402) Requires reductions in the maximum limits for out-of-pocket expenses for individuals enrolled in qualified health plans whose incomes are between 100% and 400% of the poverty line.

Subpart B: Eligibility Determinations
(Sec. 1411) Requires the Secretary to establish a program for verifying the eligibility of applicants for participation in a qualified health plan offered through an Exchange or for a tax credit for premium assistance based upon their income or their citizenship or immigration status. Requires an Exchange to submit information received from an applicant to the Secretary for verification of applicant eligibility. Provides for confidentiality of applicant information and for

an appeals and redetermination process for denials of eligibility. Imposes civil penalties on applicants for providing false or fraudulent information relating to eligibility.

Requires the Secretary to study and report to Congress by January 1, 2013, on procedures necessary to ensure the protection of privacy and due process rights in making eligibility and other determinations under this Act.

(Sec. 1412) Requires the Secretary to establish a program for advance payments of the tax credit for premium assistance and for reductions of cost-sharing. Prohibits any federal payments, tax credit, or cost-sharing reductions for individuals who are not lawfully present in the United States.

(Sec. 1413) Requires the Secretary to establish a system to enroll state residents who apply to an Exchange in state health subsidy programs, including Medicaid or the Children's Health Insurance Program (CHIP, formerly known as SCHIP), if such residents are found to be eligible for such programs after screening.

(Sec. 1414) Requires the Secretary of the Treasury to disclose to HHS personnel certain taxpayer information to determine eligibility for programs under this Act or certain other social security programs.

(Sec. 1415) Disregards the premium assistance tax credit and cost-sharing reductions in determining eligibility for federal and federally-assisted programs.

(Sec. 1416, as added by section 10105) Directs the HHS Secretary to study and report to Congress by January 1, 2013, on the feasibility and implication of adjusting the application of the federal poverty level under this subtitle for different geographic areas in the United States, including its territories.

Part II: Small Business Tax Credit

(Sec. 1421, as modified by section 10105) Allows qualified small employers to elect, beginning in 2010, a tax credit for 50% of their employee health care coverage expenses. Defines "qualified small employer" as an employer who has no more than 25 employees with average annual compensation levels not exceeding $50,000. Requires a phase-out of such credit based on employer size and employee compensation.

Subtitle F: Shared Responsibility for Health Care

Part I: Individual Responsibility

(Sec. 1501, as modified by section 10106) Requires individuals to maintain minimal essential health care coverage beginning in 2014. Imposes a penalty for failure to maintain such coverage beginning in 2014, except for certain low-income individuals who cannot afford coverage, members of Indian tribes, and individuals who suffer hardship. Exempts from the coverage requirement individuals who object to health care coverage on religious grounds, individuals not lawfully present in the United States, and individuals who are incarcerated.

(Sec. 1502) Requires providers of minimum essential coverage to file informational returns providing identifying information of covered individuals and the dates of coverage. Requires the IRS to send a notice to taxpayers who are not enrolled in minimum essential coverage about services available through the Exchange operating in their state.

Part II: Employer Responsibilities

(Sec. 1511) Amends the Fair Labor Standards Act of 1938 to: (1) require employers with more than 200 full-time employees to automatically enroll new employees in a health care plan and provide notice of the opportunity to opt-out of such coverage; and (2) provide notice to employees about an Exchange, the availability of a tax credit for premium assistance, and the loss of an employer's contribution to an employer-provided health benefit plan if the employee purchases a plan through an Exchange.

(Sec. 1513, as modified by section 10106) Imposes fines on large employers (employers with more than 50 full-time employees) who fail to offer their full-time employees the opportunity to enroll in minimum essential coverage or who have a waiting period for enrollment of more than 60 days.

Requires the Secretary of Labor to study and report to Congress on whether employees' wages are reduced due to fines imposed on employers.

(Sec. 1514, as modified by section 10106) Requires large employers to file a report with the Secretary of the Treasury on health insurance coverage provided to their full-time employees. Requires such reports to contain: (1) a certification as to whether such employers provide their full-time employees (and their dependents) the opportunity to enroll in minimum essential coverage under an eligible employer-sponsored plan; (2) the length of any waiting period for such coverage; (3) the months during which such coverage was available; (4) the monthly premium for the lowest cost option in each of the enrollment categories under the plan; (5) the employer's share of the total allowed costs of benefits provided under the plan; and (6) identifying information about the employer and full-time employees. Imposes a penalty on employers who fail to provide such report. Authorizes the Secretary of the Treasury to review the accuracy of information provided by large employers.

(Sec. 1515) Allows certain small employers to include as a benefit in a tax-exempt cafeteria plan a qualified health plan offered through an Exchange.

Subtitle G: Miscellaneous Provisions

(Sec. 1551) Applies the definitions under the Public Health Service Act related to health insurance coverage to this title.

(Sec. 1552) Requires the HHS Secretary to publish on the HHS website a list of all of the authorities provided to the Secretary under this Act.

(Sec. 1553) Prohibits the federal government, any state or local government or health care provider that receives federal financial assistance under this Act, or any health plan created under this Act, from discriminating against an individual or institutional health care entity on the basis that such individual or entity does not provide a health care item or service furnished for the purpose of causing, or assisting in causing, the death of any individual, such as by assisted suicide, euthanasia, or mercy killing.

(Sec. 1554) Prohibits the Secretary from promulgating any regulation that: (1) creates an unreasonable barrier to the ability of individuals to obtain appropriate medical care; (2) impedes timely access to health care services; (3) interferes with communications regarding a full range of treatment options between the patient and the health care provider; (4) restricts the ability of health care providers to provide full disclosure of all relevant information to patients making health care decisions; (5) violates the principle of informed consent and the ethical standards of health care professionals; or (6) limits the availability of health care treatment for the full duration of a patient's medical needs.

(Sec. 1555) Declares that no individual, company, business, nonprofit entity, or health insurance issuer offering group or individual health insurance coverage shall be required to participate in any federal health insurance program created by or expanded under this Act. Prohibits any penalty from being imposed upon any such issuer for choosing not to participate in any such program.

(Sec. 1556) Amends the Black Lung Benefits Act, with respect to claims filed on or after the effective date of the Black Lung Benefits Amendments of 1981, to eliminate exceptions to: (1) the applicability of certain provisions regarding rebuttable presumptions; and (2) the prohibition against requiring eligible survivors of a miner determined to be eligible for black lung benefits to file a new claim or to refile or otherwise revalidate the miner's claim.

(Sec. 1557) Prohibits discrimination by any federal health program or activity on the grounds of race, color, national origin, sex, age, or disability.

(Sec. 1558) Amends the Fair Labor Standards Act of 1938 to prohibit an employer from discharging or discriminating against any employee because the employee: (1) has received a health insurance credit or subsidy; (2) provides information relating to any violation of any provision of such Act; or (3) objects to, or refuses to participate in, any activity, policy, practice, or assigned task that the employee reasonably believed to be in violation of such Act.

(Sec. 1559) Gives the HHS Inspector General oversight authority with respect to the administration and implementation of this title.

(Sec. 1560) Declares that nothing in this title shall be construed to modify, impair, or supersede the operation of any antitrust laws.

(Sec. 1561) Amends the Public Health Service Act to require the Secretary to: (1) develop interoperable and secure standards and protocols that facilitate enrollment of individuals in federal and state health and human services programs; and (2) award grants to develop and adapt technology systems to implement such standards and protocols.

(Sec. 1562, as added by Sec. 10107) Directs the Comptroller General to study denials by health plans of coverage for medical services and of applications to enroll in health insurance.

(Sec. 1563, as added by Sec. 10107) Disallows the waiver of laws or regulations establishing procurement requirements relating to small business concerns with respect to any contract awarded under any program or other authority under this Act.

(Sec. 1563 [sic], as modified by Sec. 10107) Makes technical and conforming amendments.

(Sec. 1563 [sic]) Expresses the sense of the Senate that: (1) the additional surplus in the Social Security Trust Fund generated by this Act should be reserved for Social Security; and (2) the net savings generated by the CLASS program (established under Title VIII of this Act) should be reserved for such program.

Title II: Role of Public Programs

Subtitle A: Improved Access to Medicaid

(Sec. 2001, as modified by Sec. 10201) Amends title XIX (Medicaid) of the SSA to extend Medicaid coverage, beginning in calendar 2014, to individuals under age 65 who are not entitled to or enrolled in Medicare and have incomes at or below 133% of the federal poverty line. Grants a state the option to expand Medicaid eligibility to such individuals as early as April 1, 2010. Provides that, for between 2014 and 2016, the federal government will pay 100% of the cost of covering newly-eligible individuals.

Increases the federal medical assistance percentage (FMAP): (1) with respect to newly eligible individuals; and (2) between January 1, 2014, and December 31, 2016, for states meeting certain eligibility requirements.

Requires Medicaid benchmark benefits to include coverage of prescription drugs and mental health services.

Grants states the option to extend Medicaid coverage to individuals who have incomes that exceed 133% of the federal poverty line beginning January 1, 2014.

(Sec. 2002) Requires a state to use an individual's or household's modified gross income to determine income eligibility for Medicaid for non-elderly individuals, without applying any income or expense disallowances, or any assets or resources test.

Exempts from this requirement: (1) individuals eligible for Medicaid through another program; (2) the elderly or Social Security Disability Insurance (SSDI) program beneficiaries; (3) the medically needy; (4) enrollees in a Medicare Savings Program; and (5) the disabled.

(Sec. 2003) Revises state authority to offer a premium assistance subsidy for qualified employer-sponsored coverage to children under age 19 to extend such a subsidy to all individuals, regardless of age.

Prohibits a state from requiring, as a condition of Medicaid eligibility, that an individual (or the individual's parent) apply for enrollment in qualified employer-sponsored coverage.

(Sec. 2004, as modified by Sec. 10201) Extends Medicaid coverage to former foster care children who are under 26 years of age.

(Sec. 2005, as modified by Sec. 10201) Revises requirements for Medicaid payments to territories, including an increase in the limits on payments for FY2011 and thereafter.

(Sec. 2006, as modified by Sec. 10201) Prescribes an adjustment to the FMAP determination for certain states recovering from a major disaster.

(Sec. 2007) Rescinds any unobligated amounts available to the Medicaid Improvement Fund for FY2014-FY2018.

Subtitle B: Enhanced Support for the Children's Health Insurance Program

(Sec. 2101, as modified by Sec. 10201) Amends SSA title XXI (State Children's Health Insurance Program) (CHIP, formerly known as SCHIP) to increase the FY2016-FY2019 enhanced FMAP for states, subject to a 100% cap.

Prohibits states from applying, before the end of FY2019, CHIP eligibility standards that are more restrictive than those under this Act.

Deems ineligible for CHIP any targeted low-income children who cannot enroll in CHIP because allotments are capped, but who are therefore eligible for tax credits in the Exchanges.

Requires the Secretary to: (1) review benefits offered for children, and related cost-sharing imposed, by qualified health plans offered through an Exchange; and (2) certify those plans whose benefits and cost-sharing are at least comparable to those provided under the particular state's CHIP plan.

Prohibits enrollment bonus payments for children enrolled in CHIP after FY2013.

Requires a state CHIP plan, beginning January 1, 2014, to use modified gross income and household income to determine CHIP eligibility.

Requires a state to treat as a targeted low-income child eligible for CHIP any child determined ineligible for Medicaid as a result of the elimination of an income disregard based on expense or type of income.

(Sec. 2102) Makes technical corrections to the Children's Health Insurance Program Reauthorization Act of 2009 (CHIPRA).

Subtitle C: Medicaid and CHIP Enrollment Simplification

(Sec. 2201) Amends SSA title XIX (Medicaid) to require enrollment application simplification and coordination with state health insurance Exchanges and CHIP via state-run websites.

(Sec. 2202) Permits hospitals to provide Medicaid services during a period of presumptive eligibility to members of all Medicaid eligibility categories.

Subtitle D: Improvements to Medicaid Services

(Sec. 2301) Requires Medicaid coverage of: (1) freestanding birth center services; and (2) concurrent care for children receiving hospice care.

(Sec. 2303) Gives states the option of extending Medicaid coverage to family planning services and supplies under a presumptive eligibility period for a categorically needy group of individuals.

Subtitle E: New Options for States
to Provide Long-Term Services and Supports

(Sec. 2401) Authorizes states to offer home and community-based attendant services and supports to Medicaid beneficiaries with disabilities who would otherwise require care in a hospital, nursing facility, intermediate care facility for the mentally retarded, or an institution for mental diseases.

(Sec. 2402) Gives states the option of: (1) providing home and community-based services to individuals eligible for services under a waiver; and (2) offering home and community-based services to specific, targeted populations.

Creates an optional eligibility category to provide full Medicaid benefits to individuals receiving home and community-based services under a state plan amendment.

(Sec. 2403) Amends the Deficit Reduction Act of 2005 to: (1) extend through FY2016 the Money Follows the Person Rebalancing Demonstration; and (2) reduce to 90 days the institutional residency period.

(Sec. 2404) Applies Medicaid eligibility criteria to recipients of home and community-based services, during calendar 2014 through 2019, in such a way as to protect against spousal impoverishment.

(Sec. 2405) Makes appropriations for FY2010-FY2014 to the Secretary, acting through the Assistant Secretary for Aging, to expand state aging and disability resource centers.

(Sec. 2406) Expresses the sense of the Senate that: (1) during the 111th session of Congress, Congress should address long-term services and supports in a comprehensive way that guarantees elderly and disabled individuals the care they need; and (2) long-term services and supports should be made available in the community in addition to institutions.

Subtitle F: Medicaid Prescription Drug Coverage

(Sec. 2501) Amends SSA title XIX (Medicaid) to: (1) increase the minimum rebate percentage for single source drugs and innovator multiple source drugs; (2)

increase the rebate for other drugs; (3) require contracts with Medicaid managed care organizations to extend prescription drug rebates (discounts) to their enrollees; (4) provide an additional rebate for new formulations of existing drugs; and (5) set a maximum rebate amount.

(Sec. 2502) Eliminates the exclusion from Medicaid coverage of, thereby extending coverage to, certain drugs used to promote smoking cessation, as well as barbiturates and benzodiazepines.

(Sec. 2503) Revises requirements with respect to pharmacy reimbursements.

Subtitle G: Medicaid Disproportionate Share Hospital (DSH) Payments

(Sec. 2551, as modified by Sec. 10201) Reduces state disproportionate share hospital (DSH) allotments, except for Hawaii, by 50% or 35% once a state's uninsurance rate decreases by 45%, depending on whether they have spent at least or more than 99.9% of their allotments on average during FY2004-FY2008. Requires a reduction of only 25% or 17.5% for low DSH states, depending on whether they have spent at least or more than 99.9% of their allotments on average during FY2004-FY2008. Prescribes allotment reduction requirements for subsequent fiscal years.

Revises DSH allotments for Hawaii for the last three quarters of FY2012, and for FY2013 and succeeding fiscal years.

Subtitle H: Improved Coordination for Dual Eligible Beneficiaries

(Sec. 2601) Declares that any Medicaid waiver for individuals dually eligible for both Medicaid and Medicare may be conducted for a period of five years, with a five-year extension, upon state request, unless the Secretary determines otherwise for specified reasons.

(Sec. 2602) Directs the Secretary to establish a Federal Coordinated Health Care Office to bring together officers and employees of the Medicare and Medicaid programs at the Centers for Medicare and Medicaid Services (CMMS) to: (1) integrate Medicaid and Medicare benefits more effectively; and (2) improve the coordination between the federal government and states for dual eligible individuals to ensure that they get full access to the items and services to which they are entitled.

Subtitle I: Improving the Quality of Medicaid for Patients and Providers

(Sec. 2701) Amends SSA title XI, as modified by CHIPRA, to direct the Secretary to: (1) identify and publish a recommended core set of adult health quality measures for Medicaid eligible adults; and (2) establish a Medicaid Quality Measurement Program.

(Sec. 2702) Requires the Secretary to identify current state practices that prohibit payment for health care-acquired conditions and to incorporate them, or elements of them, which are appropriate for application in regulations to the Medicaid program. Requires such regulations to prohibit payments to states for any amounts expended for providing medical assistance for specified health care-acquired conditions.

(Sec. 2703) Gives states the option to provide coordinated care through a health home for individuals with chronic conditions. Authorizes the Secretary to award planning grants to states to develop a state plan amendment to that effect.

(Sec. 2704) Directs the Secretary to establish a demonstration project to evaluate the use of bundled payments for the provision of integrated care for a Medicaid beneficiary: (1) with respect to an episode of care that includes a hospitalization; and (2) for concurrent physicians services provided during a hospitalization.

(Sec. 2705) Requires the Secretary to establish a Medicaid Global Payment System Demonstration Project under which a participating state shall adjust payments made to an eligible safety net hospital or network from a fee-for-service payment structure to a global capitated payment model. Authorizes appropriations.

(Sec. 2706) Directs the Secretary to establish the Pediatric Accountable Care Organization Demonstration Project to authorize a participating state to allow pediatric medical providers meeting specified requirements to be recognized as an accountable care organization for the purpose of receiving specified incentive payments. Authorizes appropriations.

(Sec. 2707) Requires the Secretary to establish a three-year Medicaid emergency psychiatric demonstration project. Makes appropriations for FY2011.

Subtitle J: Improvements to the Medicaid and CHIP Payment and Access Commission (MACPAC)

(Sec. 2801) Revises requirements with respect to the Medicaid and CHIP Payment and Access Commission (MACPAC) and the Medicare Payment Advisory Commission (MEDPAC), including those for MACPAC membership, topics to be reviewed, and MEDPAC review of Medicaid trends in spending, utilization, and financial performance.

Requires MACPAC and MEDPAC to consult with one another on related issues.

Makes appropriations to MACPAC for FY2010.

Subtitle K: Protections for American Indians and Alaska Natives

(Sec. 2901) Sets forth special rules relating to Indians.

Declares that health programs operated by the Indian Health Service (IHS), Indian tribes, tribal organizations, and Urban Indian organizations shall be the payer of last resort for services they provide to eligible individuals.

Makes such organizations Express Lane agencies for determining Medicaid and CHIP eligibility.

(Sec. 2902) Makes permanent the requirement that the Secretary reimburse certain Indian hospitals and clinics for all Medicare Part B services.

Subtitle L: Maternal and Child Health Services

(Sec. 2951) Amends SSA title V (Maternal and Child Health Services) to direct the Secretary to make grants to eligible entities for early childhood home visitation programs. Makes appropriations for FY2010-FY2014.

(Sec. 2952) Encourages the Secretary to continue activities on postpartum depression or postpartum psychosis, including research to expand the understanding of their causes and treatment.

Authorizes the Secretary to make grants to eligible entities for projects to establish, operate, and coordinate effective and cost-efficient systems for the delivery of essential services to individuals with or at risk for postpartum conditions and their families. Authorizes appropriations for FY2010-FY2012.

(Sec. 2953, as modified by Sec. 10201) Directs the Secretary to allot funds to states to award grants to local organizations and other specified entities to carry out personal responsibility education programs to educate adolescents on both abstinence and contraception for the prevention of pregnancy and sexually transmitted infections, as well as on certain adulthood preparation subjects. Makes appropriations for FY2010-FY2014.

(Sec. 2954) Makes appropriations for FY2010-FY2014 for abstinence education.

(Sec. 2955) Requires the case review system for children aging out of foster care and independent living programs to include information about the importance of having a health care power of attorney in transition planning.

Title III: Improving the Quality and Efficiency of Health Care

Subtitle A: Transforming the Health Care Delivery System

Part I: Linking Payment to Quality Outcomes under the Medicare Program

(Sec. 3001) Amends SSA title XVIII (Medicare) to direct the Secretary to establish a hospital value-based purchasing program under which value-based incentive payments are made in a fiscal year to hospitals that meet specified performance standards for a certain performance period.

Directs the Secretary to establish value-based purchasing demonstration programs for: (1) inpatient critical access hospital services; and (2) hospitals excluded from the program because of insufficient numbers of measures and cases.

(Sec. 3002) Extends through 2013 the authority for incentive payments under the physician quality reporting system. Prescribes an incentive (penalty) for providers who do not report quality measures satisfactorily, beginning in 2015.

Requires the Secretary to integrate reporting on quality measures with reporting requirements for the meaningful use of electronic health records.

(Sec. 3003) Requires specified new types of reports and data analysis under the physician feedback program.

(Sec. 3004) Requires long-term care hospitals, inpatient rehabilitation hospitals, and hospices, starting in rate year 2014, to submit data on specified quality measures. Requires reduction of the annual update of entities which do not comply.

(Sec. 3005) Directs the Secretary, starting FY2014, to establish quality reporting programs for inpatient cancer hospitals exempt from the prospective payment system.

(Sec. 3006, as modified by Sec. 10301) Directs the Secretary to develop a plan to implement value-based purchasing programs for Medicare payments for skilled nursing facilities (SNFs), home health agencies, and ambulatory surgical centers.

(Sec. 3007) Directs the Secretary to establish a value-based payment modifier, under the physician fee schedule, based upon the quality of care furnished compared to cost.

(Sec. 3008) Subjects hospitals to a penalty adjustment to hospital payments for high rates of hospital-acquired conditions.

Part II: National Strategy to Improve Health Care Quality

(Sec. 3011, as modified by Sec. 10302) Amends the Public Health Service Act to direct the Secretary, through a transparent collaborative process, to establish a National Strategy for Quality Improvement in health care services, patient health outcomes, and population health, taking into consideration certain limitations on the use of comparative effectiveness data.

(Sec. 3012) Directs the President to convene an Interagency Working Group on Health Care Quality.

(Sec. 3013, as modified by Sec. 10303) Directs the Secretary, at least triennially, to identify gaps where no quality measures exist as well as existing quality measures that need improvement, updating, or expansion, consistent with the national strategy for use in federal health programs.

Directs the Secretary to award grants, contracts, or intergovernmental agreements to eligible entities for purposes of developing, improving, updating, or expanding such quality measures.

Requires the Secretary to develop and update periodically provider-level outcome measures for hospitals and physicians, as well as other appropriate providers.

(Sec. 3014, as modified by Sec. 10304) Requires the convening of multistakeholder groups to provide input into the selection of quality and efficiency measures.

(Sec. 3015, as modified by Sec. 10305) Directs the Secretary to: (1) establish an overall strategic framework to carry out the public reporting of performance information; and (2) collect and aggregate consistent data on quality and resource use measures from information systems used to support health care delivery. Authorizes the Secretary to award grants for such purpose.

Directs the Secretary to make available to the public, through standardized Internet websites, performance information summarizing data on quality measures.

Part III: Encouraging Development of New Patient Care Models

(Sec. 3021, as modified by Sec. 10306) Creates within CMMS a Center for Medicare and Medicaid Innovation to test innovative payment and service delivery models to reduce program expenditures while preserving or enhancing the quality of care furnished to individuals. Makes appropriations for FY2010-FY2019.

(Sec. 3022, as modified by Sec. 10307) Directs the Secretary to establish a shared savings program that: (1) promotes accountability for a patient population; (2) coordinates items and services under Medicare Parts A and B; and (3) encourages investment in infrastructure and redesigned care processes for high quality and efficient service delivery.

(Sec. 3023, as modified by Sec. 10308) Directs the Secretary to establish a pilot program for integrated care (involving payment bundling) during an episode of care provided to an applicable beneficiary around a hospitalization in order to improve the coordination, quality, and efficiency of health care services.

(Sec. 3024) Directs the Secretary to conduct a demonstration program to test a payment incentive and service delivery model that utilizes physician and nurse practitioner directed home-based primary care teams designed to reduce expenditures and improve health outcomes in the provision of items and services to applicable beneficiaries.

(Sec. 3025, as modified by Sec. 10309) Requires the Secretary to establish a hospital readmissions reduction program involving certain payment adjustments, effective for discharges on or after October 1, 2012, for certain potentially preventable Medicare inpatient hospital readmissions.

Directs the Secretary to make available a program for hospitals with a high severity adjusted readmission rate to improve their readmission rates through the use of patient safety organizations.

(Sec. 3026) Directs the Secretary to establish a Community-Based Care Transitions Program which provides funding to eligible entities that furnish improved care transitions services to high-risk Medicare beneficiaries.

(Sec. 3027) Amends the Deficit Reduction Act of 2005 to extend certain Gainsharing Demonstration Projects through FY2011.

Subtitle B: Improving Medicare for Patients and Providers

Part 1: Ensuring Beneficiary Access to Physician Care and Other Services

(Sec. 3102) Extends through calendar 2010 the floor on geographic indexing adjustments to the work portion of the physician fee schedule. Revises requirements for calculation of the practice expense portion of the geographic adjustment factor applied in a fee schedule area for services furnished in 2010 or 2011. Directs the Secretary to analyze current methods of establishing practice expense geographic adjustments and make appropriate further adjustments (a new methodology) to such adjustments for 2010 and subsequent years.

(Sec. 3103) Extends the process allowing exceptions to limitations on medically necessary therapy caps through December 31, 2010.

(Sec. 3104) Amends the Medicare, Medicaid, and SCHIP Benefits Improvement and Protection Act of 2000 to extend until January 1, 2010, an exception to a payment rule that permits laboratories to receive direct Medicare reimbursement when providing the technical component of certain physician pathology services that had been outsourced by certain (rural) hospitals.

(Sec. 3105, as modified by Sec. 10311) Amends SSA title XVIII (Medicare) to extend the bonus and increased payments for ground ambulance services until January 1, 2011.

Amends the Medicare Improvements for Patients and Providers Act of 2008 (MIPPA) to extend the payment of certain urban air ambulance services until January 1, 2011.

(Sec. 3106, as modified by Sec. 10312) Amends the Medicare, Medicaid, and SCHIP Extension Act of 2007, as modified by the American Recovery and Reinvestment Act, to extend for two years: (1) certain payment rules for long-term care hospital services; and (2) a certain moratorium on the establishment of certain hospitals and facilities.

(Sec. 3107) Amends MIPPA to extend the physician fee schedule mental health add-on payment provision through December 31, 2010.

(Sec. 3108) Allows a physician assistant who does not have a direct or indirect employment relationship with a SNF, but who is working in collaboration with a physician, to certify the need for post-hospital extended care services for Medicare payment purposes.

(Sec. 3109) Amends SSA title XVIII (Medicare), as modified by MIPPA, to exempt certain pharmacies from accreditation requirements until the Secretary develops pharmacy-specific standards.

(Sec. 3110) Creates a special Part B enrollment period for military retirees, their spouses (including widows/widowers), and dependent children, who are otherwise eligible for TRICARE (the health care plan under the Department of

Defense [DOD]) and entitled to Medicare Part A (Hospital Insurance) based on disability or end stage renal disease, but who have declined Medicare Part B (Supplementary Medical Insurance).

(Sec. 3111) Sets payments for dual-energy x-ray absorptiometry services in 2010 and 2011 at 70% of the 2006 reimbursement rates. Directs the Secretary to arrange with the Institute of Medicine of the National Academies to study and report to the Secretary and Congress on the ramifications of Medicare reimbursement reductions for such services on beneficiary access to bone mass measurement benefits.

(Sec. 3112) Eliminates funding in the Medicare Improvement Fund FY2014.

(Sec. 3113) Directs the Secretary to conduct a demonstration project under Medicare Part B of separate payments for complex diagnostic laboratory tests provided to individuals.

(Sec. 3114) Increases from 65% to 100% of the fee schedule amount provided for the same service performed by a physician the fee schedule for certified-midwife services provided on or after January 1, 2011.

Part II: Rural Protections

(Sec. 3121) Extends through 2010 hold harmless provisions under the prospective payment system for hospital outpatient department services.

Removes the 100-bed limitation for sole community hospitals so all such hospitals receive an 85% increase in the payment difference in 2010.

(Sec. 3122) Amends the Medicare Prescription Drug, Improvement, and Modernization Act of 2003, as modified by other federal law, to extend from July 1, 2010, until July 1, 2011, the reasonable cost reimbursement for clinical diagnostic laboratory service for qualifying rural hospitals with under 50 beds.

(Sec. 3123, as modified by Sec. 10313) Extends the Rural Community Hospital Demonstration Program for five additional years. Expands the maximum number of participating hospitals to 30, and to 20 the number of demonstration states with low population densities.

(Sec. 3124) Extends the Medicare-dependent Hospital Program through FY2012.

(Sec. 3125, as modified by Sec. 10314) Modifies the Medicare inpatient hospital payment adjustment for low-volume hospitals for FY2011-FY2012.

(Sec. 3126) Revises requirements for the Demonstration Project on Community Health Integration Models in Certain Rural Counties to allow additional counties as well as physicians to participate.

(Sec. 3127) Directs MEDPAC to study and report to Congress on the adequacy of payments for items and services furnished by service providers and suppliers in rural areas under the Medicare program.

(Sec. 3128) Allows a critical access hospital to continue to be eligible to receive 101% of reasonable costs for providing: (1) outpatient care regardless of the eligible billing method such hospital uses; and (2) qualifying ambulance services.

(Sec. 3129) Extends through FY2012 FLEX grants under the Medicare Rural Hospital Flexibility Program. Allows the use of grant funding to assist small rural hospitals to participate in delivery system reforms.

Part III: Improving Payment Accuracy

(Sec. 3131, as modified by Sec. 10315) Requires the Secretary, starting in 2014, to rebase home health payments by an appropriate percentage, among other things, to reflect the number, mix, and level of intensity of home health services in an episode, and the average cost of providing care.

Directs the Secretary to study and report to Congress on home health agency costs involved with providing ongoing access to care to low-income Medicare beneficiaries or beneficiaries in medically underserved areas, and in treating beneficiaries with varying levels of severity of illness. Authorizes a Medicare demonstration project based on the study results.

(Sec. 3132) Requires the Secretary, by January 1, 2011, to begin collecting additional data and information needed to revise payments for hospice care.

Directs the Secretary, not earlier than October 1, 2013, to implement, by regulation, budget neutral revisions to the methodology for determining hospice payments for routine home care and other services, which may include per diem payments reflecting changes in resource intensity in providing such care and services during the course of an entire episode of hospice care.

Requires the Secretary to impose new requirements on hospice providers participating in Medicare, including requirements for: (1) a hospice physician or nurse practitioner to have a face-to-face encounter with the individual regarding eligibility and recertification; and (2) a medical review of any stays exceeding 180 days, where the number of such cases exceeds a specified percentage of them for all hospice programs.

(Sec. 3133, as modified by Sec. 10316) Specifies reductions to Medicare DSH payments for FY2015 and ensuing fiscal years, especially to subsection (d) hospitals, to reflect lower uncompensated care costs relative to increases in the number of insured. (Generally, a subsection [d] hospital is an acute care hospital, particularly one that receives payments under Medicare's inpatient prospective payment system when providing covered inpatient services to eligible beneficiaries.)

(Sec. 3134) Directs the Secretary periodically to identify physician services as being potentially misvalued, and make appropriate adjustments to the relative values of such services under the Medicare physician fee schedule.

(Sec. 3135) Increases the presumed utilization rate for calculating the payment for advanced imaging equipment other than low-tech imaging such as ultrasound, x-rays and EKGs.

Increases the technical component payment "discount" for sequential imaging services on contiguous body parts during the same visit.

(Sec. 3136) Restricts the lump-sum payment option for new or replacement chairs to the complex, rehabilitative power-driven wheelchairs only. Eliminates the lump-sum payment option for all other power-driven wheelchairs. Makes the rental payment for power-driven wheelchairs 15% of the purchase price for each of the first three months (instead of 10%), and 6% of the purchase price for each of the remaining 10 months of the rental period (instead of 7.5%).

(Sec. 3137, as modified by Sec. 10317) Amends the Tax Relief and Health Care Act of 2006, as modified by other federal law, to extend "Section 508" hospital reclassifications until September 30, 2010, with a special rule for FY2010. ("Section 508" refers to Section 508 of the Medicare Modernization Act of 2003, which allows the temporary reclassification of a hospital with a low Medicare area wage index, for reimbursement purposes, to a nearby location with a higher Medicare area wage index, so that the "Section 508 hospital" will receive the higher Medicare reimbursement rate.)

Directs the Secretary to report to Congress a plan to reform the hospital wage index system.

(Sec. 3138) Requires the Secretary to determine if the outpatient costs incurred by inpatient prospective payment system-exempt cancer hospitals, including those for drugs and biologics, with respect to Medicare ambulatory payment classification groups, exceed those costs incurred by other hospitals reimbursed under the outpatient prospective payment system (OPPS). Requires the Secretary, if this is so, to provide for an appropriate OPPS adjustment to reflect such higher costs for services furnished on or after January 1, 2011.

(Sec. 3139) Allows a biosimilar biological product to be reimbursed at 6% of the average sales price of the brand biological product.

(Sec. 3140) Directs the Secretary to establish a Medicare Hospice Concurrent Care demonstration program under which Medicare beneficiaries are furnished, during the same period, hospice care and any other Medicare items or services from Medicare funds otherwise paid to such hospice programs.

(Sec. 3141) Requires application of the budget neutrality requirement associated with the effect of the imputed rural floor on the area wage index under the Balanced Budget Act of 1997 through a uniform national, instead of state-by-state, adjustment to the area hospital wage index floor.

(Sec. 3142) Directs the Secretary to study and report to Congress on the need for an additional payment for urban Medicare-dependent hospitals for inpatient hospital services under Medicare.

(Sec. 3143) Declares that nothing in this Act shall result in the reduction of guaranteed home health benefits under the Medicare program.

Subtitle C: Provisions Relating to Part C

(Sec. 3201, as modified by Sec. 10318) Bases the Medicare Advantage (MA) benchmark on the average of the bids from MA plans in each market.

Revises the formula for calculating the annual Medicare+Choice capitation rate to reduce the national MA per capita Medicare+Choice growth percentage used to increase benchmarks in 2011.

Increases the monthly MA plan rebates from 75% to 100% of the average per capita savings.

Requires that bid information which MA plans are required to submit to the Secretary be certified by a member of the American Academy of Actuaries and meet actuarial guidelines and rules established by the Secretary.

Directs the Secretary, acting through the CMMS Chief Actuary, to establish actuarial guidelines for the submission of bid information and bidding rules that are appropriate to ensure accurate bids and fair competition among MA plans.

Directs the Secretary to: (1) establish new MA payment areas for urban areas based on the Core Based Statistical Area; and (2) make monthly care coordination and management performance bonus payments, quality performance bonus payments, and quality bonuses for new and low enrollment MA plans, to MA plans that meet certain criteria.

Directs the Secretary to provide transitional rebates for the provision of extra benefits to enrollees.

(Sec. 3202) Prohibits MA plans from charging beneficiaries cost sharing for chemotherapy administration services, renal dialysis services, or skilled nursing care that is greater than what is charged under the traditional fee-for-service program.

Requires MA plans to apply the full amount of rebates, bonuses, and supplemental premiums according to the following order: (1) reduction of cost sharing, (2) coverage of preventive care and wellness benefits, and (3) other benefits not covered under the original Medicare fee-for-service program.

(Sec. 3203) Requires the Secretary to analyze the differences in coding patterns between MA and the original Medicare fee-for-service programs. Authorizes the Secretary to incorporate the results of the analysis into risk scores for 2014 and subsequent years.

(Sec. 3204) Allows beneficiaries to disenroll from an MA plan and return to the traditional Medicare fee-for-service program from January 1 to March 15 of each year.

Revises requirements for annual beneficiary election periods.

(Sec. 3205) Amends SSA title XVIII (Medicare), as modified by MIPPA, to extend special needs plan (SNP) authority through December 31, 2013.

Authorizes the Secretary to establish a frailty payment adjustment under PACE payment rules for fully-integrated, dual-eligible SNPs.

Extends authority through calendar 2012 for SNPs that do not have contracts with state Medicaid programs to continue to operate, but not to expand their service areas.

Directs the Secretary to require an MA organization offering a specialized MA plan for special needs individuals to be approved by the National Committee for Quality Assurance.

Requires the Secretary to use a risk score reflecting the known underlying risk profile and chronic health status of similar individuals, instead of the default risk score, for new enrollees in MA plans that are not specialized MA SNPs.

(Sec. 3206) Extends through calendar 2012 the length of time reasonable cost plans may continue operating regardless of any other MA plans serving the area.

(Sec. 3208) Creates a new type of MA plan called an MA Senior Housing Facility Plan, which would be allowed to limit its service area to a senior housing facility (continuing care retirement community) within a geographic area.

(Sec. 3209) Declares that the Secretary is not required to accept any or every bid submitted by an MA plan or Medicare Part D prescription drug plan that proposes to increase significantly any beneficiary cost sharing or decrease benefits offered.

(Sec. 3210) Directs the Secretary to request the National Association of Insurance Commissioners (NAIC) to develop new standards for certain Medigap plans.

Subtitle D: Medicare Part D Improvements for Prescription Drug Plans and MA-PD Plans

(Sec. 3301) Amends Medicare Part D (Voluntary Prescription Drug Benefit Program) to establish conditions for the availability of coverage for Part D drugs. Requires the manufacturer to participate in the Medicare coverage gap discount program.

Directs the Secretary to establish such a program.

(Sec. 3302) Excludes the MA rebate amounts and quality bonus payments from calculation of the regional low-income subsidy benchmark premium for MA monthly prescription drug beneficiaries.

(Sec. 3303) Directs the Secretary to permit a prescription drug plan or an MA-PD plan to waive the monthly beneficiary premium for a subsidy eligible individual if the amount of such premium is *de minimis*. Provides that, if such premium is waived, the Secretary shall not reassign subsidy eligible individuals enrolled in the plan to other plans based on the fact that the monthly beneficiary premium under the plan was greater than the low-income benchmark premium amount.

Authorizes the Secretary to auto-enroll subsidy eligible individuals in plans that waive *de minimis* premiums.

(Sec. 3304) Sets forth a special rule for widows and widowers regarding eligibility for low-income assistance. Allows the surviving spouse of an eligible couple to delay redetermination of eligibility for one year after the death of a spouse.

(Sec. 3305) Directs the Secretary, in the case of a subsidy eligible individual enrolled in one prescription drug plan but subsequently reassigned by the Secretary to a new prescription drug plan, to provide the individual with: (1) information on formulary differences between the individual's former plan and the new plan with respect to the individual's drug regimens; and (2) a description of the individual's right to request a coverage determination, exception, or reconsideration, bring an appeal, or resolve a grievance.

(Sec. 3306) Amends MIPPA to provide additional funding for FY2010-FY2012 for outreach and education activities related to specified Medicare low-income assistance programs.

(Sec. 3307) Authorizes the Secretary to identify classes of clinical concern through rulemaking, including anticonvulsants, antidepressants, antineoplastics, antipsychotics, antiretrovirals, and immunosuppressants for the treatment of transplant rejection. Requires prescription drug plan sponsors to include all drugs in these classes in their formularies.

(Sec. 3308) Requires Part D enrollees who exceed certain income thresholds to pay higher premiums. Revises the current authority of the IRS to disclose income information to the Social Security Administration for purposes of adjusting the Part B subsidy.

(Sec. 3309) Eliminates cost sharing for certain dual eligible individuals receiving care under a home and community-based waiver program who would otherwise require institutional care.

(Sec. 3310) Directs the Secretary to require sponsors of prescription drug plans to utilize specific, uniform techniques for dispensing covered Part D drugs to enrollees who reside in a long-term care facility in order to reduce waste associated with 30-day refills.

(Sec. 3311) Directs the Secretary to develop and maintain an easy to use complaint system to collect and maintain information on MA-PD plan and prescription drug complaints received by the Secretary until the complaint is resolved.

(Sec. 3312) Requires a prescription drug plan sponsor to: (1) use a single, uniform exceptions and appeals process for determination of a plan enrollee's prescription drug coverage; and (2) provide instant access to this process through a toll-free telephone number and an Internet website.

(Sec. 3313) Requires the HHS Inspector General to study and report to Congress on the inclusion in formularies of: (1) drugs commonly used by dual eligibles; and (2) prescription drug prices under Medicare Part D and Medicaid.

(Sec. 3314) Allows the costs incurred by AIDS drug assistance programs and by IHS in providing prescription drugs to count toward the annual out-of-pocket threshold.

(Sec. 3315) Increases by $500 the 2010 standard initial coverage limit (thus decreasing the time that a Part D enrollee would be in the coverage gap).

Subtitle E: Ensuring Medicare Sustainability

(Sec. 3401, as modified by Sec. 10319 and Sec. 10322) Revises certain market basket updates and incorporates a full productivity adjustment into any updates that do not already incorporate such adjustments, including inpatient hospitals, home health providers, nursing homes, hospice providers, inpatient psychiatric facilities, long-term care hospitals, inpatient rehabilitation facilities, and Part B providers.

Establishes a quality measure reporting program for psychiatric hospitals beginning in FY2014.

(Sec. 3402) Revises requirements for reduction of the Medicare Part B premium subsidy based on income. Maintains the current 2010 income thresholds for the period of 2011 through 2019.

(Sec. 3403, as modified by Sec. 10320) Establishes an Independent Medicare Advisory Board to develop and submit detailed proposals to reduce the per capita rate of growth in Medicare spending to the President for the Congress to consider. Establishes a consumer advisory council to advise the Board on the impact of payment policies under this title on consumers.

Subtitle F: Health Care Quality Improvements

(Sec. 3501) Amends the Public Health Service Act to direct the Center for Quality Improvement and Patient Safety of the Agency for Healthcare Research and Quality (AHRQ) to conduct or support activities for best practices in the delivery of health care services and support research on the development of tools to facilitate adoption of best practices that improve the quality, safety, and efficiency of health care delivery services. Authorizes appropriations for FY2010–FY2014.

Requires the AHRQ Director, through the AHRQ Center for Quality Improvement and Patient Safety, to award grants or contracts to eligible entities to provide technical support or to implement models and practices identified in the research conducted by the Center.

(Sec. 3502, as modified by Sec. 10321) Directs the Secretary to establish a program to provide grants to or enter into contracts with eligible entities to establish community-based interdisciplinary, interprofessional teams to support primary care practices, including obstetrics and gynecology practices, within the hospital service areas served by the eligible entities.

(Sec. 3503) Directs the Secretary, acting through the Patient Safety Research Center, to establish a program to provide grants or contracts to eligible entities to implement medication management services provided by licensed pharmacists, as a collaborative multidisciplinary, inter-professional approach to the treatment of chronic diseases for targeted individuals, to improve the quality of care and reduce overall cost in the treatment of such disease.

(Sec. 3504) Directs the Secretary, acting through the Assistant Secretary for Preparedness and Response, to award at least four multiyear contracts or competitive grants to eligible entities to support pilot projects that design, implement, and evaluate innovative models of regionalized, comprehensive, and accountable emergency care and trauma systems.

Requires the Secretary to support federal programs administered by the National Institutes of Health, the AHRQ, the Health Resources and Services Administration (HRSA), the CMMS, and other agencies involved in improving the emergency care system to expand and accelerate research in emergency medical care systems and emergency medicine.

Directs the Secretary to support federal programs administered by the such agencies to coordinate and expand research in pediatric emergency medical care systems and pediatric emergency medicine.

Authorizes appropriations for FY2010-FY2014.

(Sec. 3505) Requires the Secretary to establish three programs to award grants to qualified public, nonprofit IHS, Indian tribal, and urban Indian trauma centers to: (1) assist in defraying substantial uncompensated care costs; (2) further the core missions of such trauma centers, including by addressing costs associated with patient stabilization and transfer; and (3) provide emergency relief to ensure the continued and future availability of trauma services. Authorizes appropriations for FY2010-FY2015.

Directs the Secretary to provide funding to states to enable them to award grants to eligible entities for trauma services. Authorizes appropriations for FY2010-FY2015.

(Sec. 3506) Directs the Secretary to: (1) establish a program to award grants or contracts to develop, update, and produce patient decision aids to assist health care providers and patients; (2) establish a program to provide for the phased-in development, implementation, and evaluation of shared decision making using patient decision aids to meet the objective of improving the understanding of patients of their medical treatment options; and (3) award grants for establishment and support of Shared Decisionmaking Resource Centers. Authorizes appropriations for FY2010 and subsequent fiscal years.

(Sec. 3507) Requires the Secretary, acting through the Commissioner of Food and Drugs, to determine whether the addition of quantitative summaries of the benefits and risks of prescription drugs in a standardized format to the promotional labeling or print advertising of such drugs would improve heath care decisionmaking by clinicians and patients and consumers.

(Sec. 3508) Authorizes the Secretary to award grants to eligible entities or consortia to carry out demonstration projects to develop and implement academic curricula that integrate quality improvement and patient safety in the clinical education of health professionals.

(Sec. 3509) Establishes an Office on Women's Health within the Office of the Secretary, the Office of the Director of the Centers for Disease Control and Prevention (CDC), the Office of the AHRQ Director, the Office of the Administrator of HRSA, and the Office of the Commissioner of Food and Drugs.

Authorizes appropriations for FY2010-FY2014 for all such Offices on Women's Health.

(Sec. 3510) Extends from three years to four years the duration of a patient navigator grant.

Prohibits the Secretary from awarding such a grant unless the recipient entity provides assurances that patient navigators recruited, assigned, trained, or employed using grant funds meet minimum core proficiencies tailored for the main focus or intervention of the navigator involved.

Authorizes appropriations for FY2010-FY2015.

(Sec. 3511) Authorizes appropriations to carry out this title, except where otherwise provided in the title.

(Sec. 3512, as added by Sec. 10201) Directs the Comptroller General to study and report to Congress on whether the development, recognition, or implementation of any guideline or other standards under specified provisions of this Act would result in the establishment of a new cause of action or claim.

Subtitle G: Protecting and Improving Guaranteed Medicare Benefits

(Sec. 3601) Provides that nothing in this Act shall result in a reduction of guaranteed benefits under the Medicare program.

States that savings generated for the Medicare program under this Act shall extend the solvency of the Medicare trust funds, reduce Medicare premiums and other cost-sharing for beneficiaries, and improve or expand guaranteed Medicare benefits and protect access to Medicare providers.

(Sec. 3602) Declares that nothing in this Act shall result in the reduction or elimination of any benefits guaranteed by law to participants in MA plans.

Title IV: Prevention of Chronic Disease and Improving Public Health

Subtitle A: Modernizing Disease Prevention and Public Health Systems

(Sec. 4001, as modified by Sec. 10401) Requires the President to: (1) establish the National Prevention, Health Promotion and Public Health Council; (2) establish the Advisory Group on Prevention, Health Promotion, and Integrative and Public Health; and (3) appoint the Surgeon General as Chairperson of the Council in order to develop a national prevention, health promotion, and public health strategy.

Requires the Secretary and the Comptroller General to conduct periodic reviews and evaluations of every federal disease prevention and health promotion initiative, program, and agency.

(Sec. 4002, as modified by Sec. 10401) Establishes a Prevention and Public Health Fund to provide for expanded and sustained national investment in prevention and public health programs to improve health and help restrain the rate of growth in private and public sector health care costs. Authorizes appropriations and appropriates money to such Fund.

(Sec 4003) Requires (currently, allows) the Director of AHRQ to convene the

Preventive Services Task Force to review scientific evidence related to the effectiveness, appropriateness, and cost-effectiveness of clinical preventive services for the purpose of developing recommendations for the health care community.

Requires the Director of CDC to convene an independent Community Preventive Services Task Force to review scientific evidence related to the effectiveness, appropriateness, and cost-effectiveness of community preventive interventions for the purpose of developing recommendations for individuals and organizations delivering populations-based services and other policy makers.

(Sec. 4004, as modified by Sec. 10401) Requires the Secretary to provide for the planning and implementation of a national public-private partnership for a prevention and health promotion outreach and education campaign to raise public awareness of health improvement across the life span.

Requires the Secretary, acting through the Director of CDC, to: (1) establish and implement a national science-based media campaign on health promotion and disease prevention; and (2) enter into a contract for the development and operation of a federal website personalized prevention plan tool.

Subtitle B: Increasing Access to Clinical Preventive Services

(Sec. 4101, as modified by Sec. 10402) Requires the Secretary to establish a program to award grants to eligible entities to support the operation of school-based health centers.

(Sec. 4102) Requires the Secretary, acting through the Director of CDC, to carry out oral health activities, including: (1) establishing a national public education campaign that is focused on oral health care prevention and education; (2) awarding demonstration grants for research-based dental caries disease management activities; (3) awarding grants for the development of school-based dental sealant programs; and (4) entering into cooperative agreements with state, territorial, and Indian tribes or tribal organizations for oral health data collection and interpretation, a delivery system for oral health, and science-based programs to improve oral health.

Requires the Secretary to: (1) update and improve the Pregnancy Risk Assessment Monitoring System as it relates to oral health care; (2) develop oral health care components for inclusion in the National Health and Nutrition Examination Survey; and (3) ensure that the Medical Expenditures Panel Survey by AHRQ includes the verification of dental utilization, expenditure, and coverage findings through conduct of a look-back analysis.

(Sec. 4103, as modified by Sec. 10402) Amends SSA title XVIII (Medicare) to provide coverage of personalized prevention plan services, including a health risk assessment, for individuals. Prohibits cost-sharing for such services.

(Sec. 4104, as modified by Sec. 10406) Eliminates cost-sharing for certain preventive services recommended by the United States Preventive Services Task Force.

(Sec. 4105) Authorizes the Secretary to modify Medicare coverage of any preventive service consistent with the recommendations of such Task Force.

(Sec. 4106) Amends SSA title XIX (Medicaid) to provide Medicaid coverage of preventive services and approved vaccines. Increases the FMAP for such services and vaccines.

(Sec. 4107) Provides for Medicaid coverage of counseling and pharmacotherapy for cessation of tobacco use by pregnant women.

(Sec. 4108) Requires the Secretary to award grants to states to carry out initiatives to provide incentives to Medicaid beneficiaries who participate in programs to lower health risk and demonstrate changes in health risk and outcomes.

Subtitle C: Creating Healthier Communities

(Sec. 4201, as modified by Sec. 10403) Requires the Secretary, acting through the Director of CDC, to award grants to state and local governmental agencies and community-based organizations for the implementation, evaluation, and dissemination of evidence-based community preventive health activities in order to reduce chronic disease rates, prevent the development of secondary conditions, address health disparities, and develop a stronger evidence base of effective prevention programming.

(Sec. 4202) Requires the Secretary, acting through the Director of CDC, to award grants to state or local health departments and Indian tribes to carry out pilot programs to provide public health community interventions, screenings, and clinical referrals for individuals who are between 55 and 64 years of age.

Requires the Secretary to: (1) conduct an evaluation of community-based prevention and wellness programs and develop a plan for promoting healthy lifestyles and chronic disease self-management for Medicare beneficiaries; and (2) evaluate community prevention and wellness programs that have demonstrated potential to help Medicare beneficiaries reduce their risk of disease, disability, and injury by making healthy lifestyle choices.

(Sec. 4203) Amends the Rehabilitation Act of 1973 to require the Architectural and Transportation Barriers Compliance Board to promulgate standards setting forth the minimum technical criteria for medical diagnostic equipment used in medical settings to ensure that such equipment is accessible to, and usable by, individuals with accessibility needs.

(Sec. 4204) Authorizes the Secretary to negotiate and enter into contracts with vaccine manufacturers for the purchase and delivery of vaccines for adults. Allows a state to purchase additional quantities of adult vaccines from manufacturers at the applicable price negotiated by the Secretary. Requires the Secretary, acting through the Director of CDC, to establish a demonstration program to award grants to states to improve the provision of recommended immunizations for children and adults through the use of evidence-based, population-based interventions for high-risk populations.

Reauthorizes appropriations for preventive health service programs to immunize children and adults against vaccine-preventable diseases without charge.

Requires the Comptroller General to study the ability of Medicare beneficiaries who are 65 years or older to access routinely recommended vaccines covered under the prescription drug program since its establishment.

(Sec. 4205) Amends the Federal Food, Drug, and Cosmetic Act to require the labeling of a food item offered for sale in a retail food establishment that is part of a chain with 20 or more locations under the same name to disclose on the menu and menu board: (1) the number of calories contained in the standard menu item; (2) the suggested daily caloric intake; and (3) the availability on the premises and upon request of specified additional nutrient information. Requires self-service facilities to place adjacent to each food offered a sign that lists calories per displayed food item or per serving. Requires vending machine operators who operate 20 or more vending machines to provide a sign disclosing the number of calories contained in each article of food.

(Sec. 4206) Requires the Secretary to establish a pilot program to test the impact of providing at-risk populations who utilize community health centers an individualized wellness plan designed to reduce risk factors for preventable conditions as identified by a comprehensive risk-factor assessment.

(Sec. 4207) Amends the Fair Labor Standards Act of 1938 to require employers to provide a reasonable break time and a suitable place, other than a bathroom, for an employee to express breast milk for her nursing child. Excludes an employer with less than 50 employees if such requirements would impose an undue hardship.

Subtitle D: Support for Prevention and Public Health Innovation

(Sec. 4301) Requires the Secretary, acting through the Director of CDC, to provide funding for research in the area of public health services and systems.

(Sec. 4302) Requires the Secretary to ensure that any federally conduced or supported health care or public health program, activity, or survey collects and reports specified demographic data regarding health disparities.

Requires the Secretary, acting through the National Coordinator for Health Information Technology, to develop: (1) national standards for the management of data collected; and (2) interoperability and security systems for data management.

(Sec. 4303, as modified by Sec. 10404) Requires the Director of CDC to: (1) provide employers with technical assistance, consultation, tools, and other resources in evaluating employer-based wellness programs; and (2) build evaluation capacity among workplace staff by training employers on how to evaluate such wellness programs and ensuring that evaluation resources, technical assistance, and consultation are available.

Requires the Director of CDC to conduct a national worksite health policies and programs survey to assess employer-based health policies and programs.

(Sec. 4304) Requires the Secretary, acting through the Director of CDC, to establish an Epidemiology and Laboratory Capacity Grant Program to award grants to assist public health agencies in improving surveillance for, and response to, infectious diseases and other conditions of public health importance.

(Sec. 4305) Requires the Secretary to: (1) enter into an agreement with the Institute of Medicine to convene a Conference on Pain, the purposes of which shall include to increase the recognition of pain as a significant public health problem in the United States; and (2) establish the Interagency Pain Research Coordinating Committee.

(Sec. 4306) Appropriates funds to carry out childhood obesity demonstration projects.

Subtitle E: Miscellaneous Provisions

(Sec. 4402) Requires the Secretary to evaluate programs to determine whether existing federal health and wellness initiatives are effective in achieving their stated goals.

Title V: Health Care Workforce

Subtitle A: Purpose and Definitions

(Sec. 5001) Declares that the purpose of this title is to improve access to and the delivery of health care services for all individuals, particularly low income, underserved, uninsured, minority, health disparity, and rural populations.

Subtitle B: Innovations in the Health Care Workforce

(Sec. 5101, as modified by Sec. 10501) Establishes a National Health Care Workforce Commission to: (1) review current and projected health care workforce supply and demand; and (2) make recommendations to Congress and the Administration concerning national health care workforce priorities, goals, and policies.

(Sec. 5102) Establishes a health care workforce development grant program.

(Sec. 5103) Requires the Secretary to establish the National Center for Health Care Workforce Analysis to provide for the development of information describing and analyzing the health care workforce and workforce related issues. Transfers the responsibilities and resources of the National Center for Health Workforce Analysis to the Center created under this section.

(Sec. 5104, as added by Sec. 10501) Establishes the Interagency Access to Health Care in Alaska Task Force to: (1) assess access to health care for beneficiaries of federal health care systems in Alaska; and (2) develop a strategy to improve delivery to such beneficiaries.

Subtitle C: Increasing the Supply of the Health Care Workforce

(Sec. 5201) Revises student loan repayment provisions related to the length of service requirement for the primary health care loan repayment program.

(Sec. 5202) Increases maximum amount of loans made by schools of nursing to students.

(Sec. 5203) Directs the Secretary to establish and carry out a pediatric specialty loan repayment program.

(Sec. 5204) Requires the Secretary to establish the Public Health Workforce Loan Repayment Program to assure an adequate supply of public health professionals to eliminate critical public health workforce shortages in federal, state, local, and tribal public health agencies.

(Sec. 5205) Amends the Higher Education Act of 1965 to expand student loan forgiveness to include allied health professionals employed in public health agencies.

(Sec. 5206) Includes public health workforce loan repayment programs as permitted activities under a grant program to increase the number of individuals in the public health workforce.

Authorizes the Secretary to provide for scholarships for mid-career professionals in the public health and allied health workforce to receive additional training in the field of public health and allied health.

(Sec. 5207) Authorizes appropriations for the National Health Service Corps Scholarship Program and the National Health Service Corps Loan Repayment Program.

(Sec. 5208) Requires the Secretary to award grants for the cost of the operation of nurse-managed health clinics.

(Sec. 5209) Eliminates the cap on the number of commissioned officers in the Public Health Service Regular Corps.

(Sec. 5210) Revises the Regular Corps and the Reserve Corps (renamed the Ready Reserve Corps) in the Public Health Service. Sets forth the uses of the Ready Reserve Corps.

Subtitle D: Enhancing Health Care Workforce Education and Training

(Sec. 5301) Sets forth provisions providing for health care professional training programs.

(Sec. 5302) Requires the Secretary to award grants for new training opportunities for direct care workers who are employed in long-term care settings.

(Sec. 5303) Sets forth provisions providing for dentistry professional training programs.

(Sec. 5304) Authorizes the Secretary to award grants for demonstration programs to establish training programs for alternative dental health care providers in order to increase access to dental health services in rural and other underserved communities.

(Sec. 5305) Requires the Secretary to award grants or contracts to entities that operate a geriatric education center to offer short-term, intensive courses that focus on geriatrics, chronic care management, and long-term care.

Expands geriatric faculty fellowship programs to make dentists eligible.

Reauthorizes and revises the geriatric education programs to allow grant funds to be used for the establishment of traineeships for individuals who are preparing for advanced education nursing degrees in areas that specialize in the care of elderly populations.

(Sec. 5306) Authorizes the Secretary to award grants to institutions of higher education to support the recruitment of students for, and education and clinical experience of the students in, social work programs, psychology programs, child and adolescent mental health, and training of paraprofessional child and adolescent mental health workers.

(Sec. 5307) Authorizes the Secretary, acting through the Administrator of HRSA, to award grants, contracts, or cooperative agreements for the development, evaluation, and dissemination of research, demonstration projects, and model curricula for health professions training in cultural competency, prevention, public health proficiency, reducing health disparities, and working with individuals with disabilities.

(Sec. 5308) Requires nurse-midwifery programs, in order to be eligible for advanced education nursing grants, to have as their objective the education of midwives and to be accredited by the American College of Nurse-Midwives Accreditation Commission for Midwifery Education.

(Sec. 5309) Authorizes the Secretary to award grants or enter into contracts to enhance the nursing workforce by initiating and maintaining nurse retention programs.

(Sec. 5310) Makes nurse faculty at an accredited school of nursing eligible for the nursing education loan repayment program.

(Sec. 5311) Revises the nurse faculty loan repayment program, including to increase the amount of such loans.

Authorizes the Secretary, acting through the Administrator of HRSA, to enter into an agreement for the repayment of education loans in exchange for service as a member of a faculty at an accredited school of nursing.

(Sec. 5312) Authorizes appropriations for carrying out nursing workforce programs.

(Sec. 5313, as modified by Sec. 10501) Requires the Director of CDC to award grants to eligible entities to promote positive health behaviors and outcomes for populations in medically underserved communities through the use of community health workers.

(Sec. 5314) Authorizes the Secretary to carry out activities to address documented workforce shortages in state and local health departments in the critical areas of applied public health epidemiology and public health laboratory science and informatics.

(Sec. 5315) Authorizes the establishment of the United States Public Health Sciences Track, which is authorized to award advanced degrees in public health, epidemiology, and emergency preparedness and response.

Directs the Surgeon General to develop: (1) an integrated longitudinal plan for health professions continuing education; and (2) faculty development programs and curricula in decentralized venues of health care to balance urban, tertiary, and inpatient venues.

(Sec. 5316, as added by Sec. 10501) Requires the Secretary to establish a training demonstration program for family nurse practitioners to employ and provide one-year training for nurse practitioners serving as primary care providers in federally qualified health centers or nurse-managed health centers.

Subtitle E: Supporting the Existing Health Care Workforce

(Sec. 5401) Revises the allocation of funds to assist schools in supporting programs of excellence in health professions education for underrepresented minority individuals and schools designated as centers of excellence.

(Sec. 5402, as modified by Sec. 10501) Makes schools offering physician assistant education programs eligible for loan repayment for health profession faculty. Increases the amount of loan repayment for such program.

Authorizes appropriations for: (1) scholarships for disadvantaged students attending health professions or nursing schools; (2) loan repayment for health professions faculty; and (3) grants to health professions school to assist individuals from disadvantaged backgrounds.

(Sec. 5403) Requires the Secretary to: (1) make awards for area health education center programs; and (2) provide for timely dissemination of research findings using relevant resources.

(Sec. 5404) Makes revisions to the grant program to increase nursing education opportunities for individuals from disadvantaged backgrounds to include providing: (1) stipends for diploma or associate degree nurses to enter a bridge or degree completion program; (2) student scholarships or stipends for accelerated nursing degree programs; and (3) advanced education preparation.

(Sec. 5405, as modified by Sec. 10501) Requires the Secretary, acting through the Director of AHRQ, to establish a Primary Care Extension Program to provide support and assistance to educate primary care providers about preventive medicine, health promotion, chronic disease management, mental and behavioral health services, and evidence-based and evidence-informed therapies and techniques.

Requires the Secretary to award grants to states for the establishment of Primary Care Extension Program State Hubs to coordinate state health care functions with quality improvement organizations and area health education centers.

Subtitle F: Strengthening Primary Care and Other Workforce Improvements

(Sec. 5501, as modified by Sec. 10501) Requires Medicare incentive payments to: (1) primary care practitioners providing primary care services on or after January 1, 2011, and before January 1, 2016; and (2) general surgeons performing major surgical procedures on or after January 1, 2011, and before January 1, 2016, in a health professional shortage area.

(Sec. 5503) Reallocates unused residency positions to qualifying hospitals for primary care residents for purposes of payments to hospitals for graduate medical education costs.

(Sec. 5504) Revises provisions related to graduate medical education costs to count the time residents spend in nonprovider settings toward the full-time equivalency if the hospital incurs the costs of the stipends and fringe benefits of such residents during such time.

(Sec. 5505, as modified by Sec. 10501) Includes toward the determination of full-time equivalency for graduate medical education costs time spent by an intern or resident in an approved medical residency training program in a nonprovider setting that is primarily engaged in furnishing patient care in nonpatient care activities.

(Sec. 5506) Directs the Secretary, when a hospital with an approved medical residency program closes, to increase the resident limit for other hospitals based on proximity criteria.

(Sec. 5507) Requires the Secretary to: (1) award grants for demonstration projects that are designed to provide certain low-income individuals with the opportunity to obtain education and training for health care occupations that pay well and that are expected to experience labor shortages or be in high demand; and (2) award grants to states to conduct demonstration projects for purposes of developing core training competencies and certification programs for personal or home care aides.

Authorizes appropriations for FY2009-FY2012 for family-to-family health information centers.

(Sec. 5508) Authorizes the Secretary to award grants to teaching health centers for the purpose of establishing new accredited or expanded primary care residency programs.

Allows up to 50% of time spent teaching by a member of the National Health

Service Corps to be considered clinical practice for purposes of fulfilling the service obligation.

Requires the Secretary to make payments for direct and indirect expenses to qualified teaching health centers for expansion or establishment of approved graduate medical residency training programs.

(Sec. 5509) Requires the Secretary to establish a graduate nurse education demonstration under which a hospital may receive payment for the hospital's reasonable costs for the provision of qualified clinical training to advance practice nurses.

Subtitle G: Improving Access to Health Care Services

(Sec. 5601) Reauthorizes appropriations for health centers to serve medically underserved populations.

(Sec. 5602) Requires the Secretary to establish through the negotiated rulemaking process a comprehensive methodology and criteria for designation of medically underserved populations and health professions shortage areas.

(Sec. 5603) Reauthorizes appropriations for FY2010-FY2014 for the expansion and improvement of emergency medical services for children who need treatment for trauma or critical care.

(Sec. 5604) Authorizes the Secretary, acting through the Administrator of the Substance Abuse and Mental Health Services Administration, to award grants and cooperative agreements for demonstration projects for the provision of coordinated and integrated services to special populations through the co-location of primary and specialty care services in community-based mental and behavioral health settings.

(Sec. 5605) Establishes a Commission on Key National Indicators to: (1) conduct comprehensive oversight of a newly established key national indicators system; and (2) make recommendations on how to improve such system. Directs the National Academy of Sciences to enable the establishment of such system by creating its own institutional capability or by partnering with an independent private nonprofit organization to implement such system. Directs the Comptroller General to study previous work conducted by all public agencies, private organizations, or foreign countries with respect to best practices for such systems.

(Sec. 5606, as added by Sec. 10501) Authorizes a state to award grants to health care providers who treat a high percentage of medically underserved populations or other special populations in the state.

Subtitle H: General Provisions

(Sec. 5701) Requires the Secretary to submit to the appropriate congressional committees a report on activities carried out under this title and the effectiveness of such activities.

Title VI: Transparency and Program Integrity

Subtitle A: Physician Ownership and Other Transparency

(Sec. 6001, as modified by Sec. 10601) Amends SSA title XVIII (Medicare) to prohibit physician-owned hospitals that do not have a provider agreement by August 1, 2010, to participate in Medicare. Allows their participation in Medicare under a rural provider and hospital exception to the ownership or investment prohibition if they meet certain requirements addressing conflict of interest, bona fide investments, patient safety issues, and expansion limitations.

(Sec. 6002) Amends SSA title XI to require drug, device, biological and medical supply manufacturers to report to the Secretary transfers of value made to a physician, physician medical practice, a physician group practice, and/or teaching hospital, as well as information on any physician ownership or investment interest in the manufacturer. Provides penalties for noncompliance. Preempts duplicative state or local laws.

(Sec. 6003) Amends SSA title XVIII (Medicare), with respect to the Medicare in-office ancillary exception to the prohibition against physician self-referrals, to require a referring physician to inform the patient in writing that the patient may obtain a specified imaging service from a person other than the referring physician, a physician who is a member of the same group practice as the referring physician, or an individual directly supervised by the physician or by another physician in the group practice. Requires the referring physician also to provide the patient with a written list of suppliers who furnish such services in the area in which the patient resides.

(Sec. 6004) Amends SSA title XI to require prescription drug manufacturers and authorized distributors of record to report to the Secretary specified information pertaining to drug samples.

(Sec. 6005) Amends SSA title XI to require a pharmacy benefit manager (PBM) or a health benefits plan that manages prescription drug coverage under a contract with a Medicare or Exchange health plan to report to the Secretary information regarding the generic dispensing rate, the rebates, discounts, or price concessions negotiated by the PBM, and the payment difference between health plans and PBMs and the PBMs and pharmacies.

Subtitle B: Nursing Home Transparency and Improvement

Part I: Improving Transparency of Information

(Sec. 6101) Amends SSA title XI to require SNFs under Medicare and nursing facilities (NFs) under Medicaid to make available, upon request by the Secretary, the HHS Inspector General, the states, or a state long-term care ombudsman, information on ownership of the SNF or NF, including a description of the facility's governing body and organizational structure, as well as information regarding additional disclosable parties.

(Sec. 6102) Requires SNFs and NFs to operate a compliance and ethics program effective in preventing and detecting criminal, civil, and administrative violations.

Directs the Secretary to establish and implement a quality assurance and performance improvement program for SNFs and NFs, including multi-unit chains of facilities.

(Sec. 6103) Amends SSA title XVIII (Medicare) to require the Secretary to publish on the Nursing Home Compare Medicare website: (1) standardized staffing data; (2) links to state Internet websites regarding state survey and certification programs; (3) the model standardized complaint form; (4) a summary of substantiated complaints; and (5) the number of adjudicated instances of criminal violations by a facility or its employee.

(Sec. 6104) Requires SNFs to report separately expenditures on wages and benefits for direct care staff, breaking out registered nurses, licensed professional nurses, certified nurse assistants, and other medical and therapy staff.

(Sec. 6105) Requires the Secretary to develop a standardized complaint form for use by residents (or a person acting on a resident's behalf) in filing complaints with a state survey and certification agency and a state long-term care ombudsman program. Requires states to to establish complaint resolution processes.

(Sec. 6106) Amends SSA title XI to require the Secretary to develop a program for facilities to report direct care staffing information on payroll and other verifiable and auditable data in a uniform format.

(Sec. 6107) Requires the Comptroller General to study and report to Congress on the Five-Star Quality Rating System for nursing homes of CMMS.

Part II: Targeting Enforcement

(Sec. 6111) Amends SSA title XVIII (Medicare) to authorize the Secretary to reduce civil monetary penalties by 50% for certain SNFs and NFs that self-report and promptly correct deficiencies within 10 calendar days of imposition of the penalty. Directs the Secretary to issue regulations providing for an informal dispute resolution process after imposition of a penalty, as well as an escrow account for money penalties pending resolution of any appeals.

(Sec. 6112) Directs the Secretary to establish a demonstration project for developing, testing, and implementing a national independent monitor program to oversee interstate and large intrastate chains of SNFs and NFs.

(Sec. 6113) Requires the administrator of a SNF or a NF that is preparing to close to notify in writing residents, legal representatives of residents or other responsible parties, the Secretary, and the state long-term care ombudsman program in advance of the closure by at least 60 days. Requires the notice to include a plan for the transfer and adequate relocation of residents to another facility or alternative setting. Requires the state to ensure a successful relocation of residents.

(Sec. 6114) Requires the Secretary to conduct two SNF-and NF-based demonstration projects to develop best practice models in two areas: (1) one for facilities involved in the "culture change" movement; and (2) one for the use of information technology to improve resident care.

Part III: Improving Staff Training

(Sec. 6121) Requires SNFs and NFs to include dementia management and abuse prevention training as part of pre-employment initial training and, if appropriate, as part of ongoing in-service training for permanent and contract or agency staff.

Subtitle C: Nationwide Program for National and State Background Checks on Direct Patient Access Employees of Long Term Care Facilities and Providers

(Sec. 6201) Requires the Secretary to establish a nationwide program for national and state background checks on prospective direct patient access employees of long-term care facilities and providers.

Subtitle D: Patient-Centered Outcomes Research

(Sec. 6301, as modified by Sec. 10602) Amends SSA title XI to establish the Patient-Centered Outcomes Research Institute to identify priorities for, and establish, update, and carry out, a national comparative outcomes research project agenda. Provides for a peer review process for primary research.

Prohibits the Institute from allowing the subsequent use of data from original research in work-for-hire contracts with individuals, entities, or instrumentalities that have a financial interest in the results, unless approved by the Institute under a data use agreement.

Amends the Public Health Service Act to direct the Office of Communication and Knowledge Transfer at AHRQ to disseminate broadly the research findings published by the Institute and other government-funded research relevant to comparative clinical effective research.

Prohibits the Secretary from using evidence and findings from Institute research to make a determination regarding Medicare coverage unless such use is through an iterative and transparent process which includes public comment and considers the effect on subpopulations.

Amends the Internal Revenue Code to establish in the Treasury the Patient-Centered Outcomes Research Trust Fund. Directs the Secretary to make transfers to that Trust Fund from the Medicare Trust Funds.

Imposes annual fees of $2 times the number of insured lives on each specified health insurance policy and on self-insured health plans.

(Sec. 6302) Terminates the Federal Coordinating Council for Comparative Effectiveness Research upon enactment of this Act.

Subtitle E: Medicare, Medicaid, and CHIP Program Integrity Provisions

(Sec. 6401, as modified by Sec. 10603) Amends SSA title XVIII (Medicare) to require the Secretary to: (1) establish procedures for screening providers and suppliers participating in Medicare, Medicaid, and CHIP; and (2) determine the level of screening according to the risk of fraud, waste, and abuse with respect to each category of provider or supplier.

Requires providers and suppliers applying for enrollment or revalidation of enrollment in Medicare, Medicaid, or CHIP to disclose current or previous affiliations with any provider or supplier that: (1) has uncollected debt; (2) has had its payments suspended; (3) has been excluded from participating in a federal health care program; or (4) has had billing privileges revoked. Authorizes the Secretary to deny enrollment in a program if these affiliations pose an undue risk to it.

Requires providers and suppliers to establish a compliance program containing specified core elements.

Directs the CMMS Administrator to establish a process for making available to each state agency with responsibility for administering a state Medicaid plan or a child health plan under SSA title XXI the identity of any provider or supplier under Medicare or CHIP who is terminated.

(Sec. 6402) Requires CMMS to include in the integrated data repository claims and payment data from Medicare, Medicaid, CHIP, and health-related programs administered by the Departments of Veterans Affairs (VA) and DOD, the Social Security Administration, and IHS.

Directs the Secretary to enter into data-sharing agreements with the Commissioner of Social Security, the VA and DOD Secretaries, and the IHS Director to help identity fraud, waste, and abuse.

Requires that overpayments be reported and returned within 60 days from the date the overpayment was identified or by the date a corresponding cost report was due, whichever is later.

Directs the Secretary to issue a regulation requiring all Medicare, Medicaid, and CHIP providers to include their National Provider Identifier on enrollment applications.

Authorizes the Secretary to withhold the federal matching payment to states for medical assistance expenditures whenever a state does not report enrollee encounter data in a timely manner to the state's Medicaid Management Information System.

Authorizes the Secretary to exclude providers and suppliers participation in any federal health care program for providing false information on any application to enroll or participate.

Subjects to civil monetary penalties excluded individuals who: (1) order or prescribe an item or service; (2) make false statements on applications or contracts to participate in a federal health care program; or (3) know of an overpayment and do not return it. Subjects the latter offense to civil monetary penalties of up to $50,000 or triple the total amount of the claim involved.

Authorizes the Secretary to issue subpoenas and require the attendance and testimony of witnesses and the production of any other evidence that relates to matters under investigation or in question.

Requires the Secretary take into account the volume of billing for a durable medical equipment (DME) supplier or home health agency when determining the size of the supplier's and agency's surety bond. Authorizes the Secretary to require other providers and suppliers to post a surety bond if the Secretary considers them to be at risk.

Authorizes the Secretary to suspend payments to a provider or supplier pending a fraud investigation.

Appropriates an additional $10 million, adjusted for inflation, to the Health Care Fraud and Abuse Control each of FY2011-FY2020. Applies inflation adjustments as well to Medicare Integrity Program funding.

Requires the Medicaid Integrity Program and Program contractors to provide the Secretary and the HHS Office of Inspector General with performance statistics, including the number and amount of overpayments recovered, the number of fraud referrals, and the return on investment for such activities.

(Sec. 6403) Requires the Secretary to furnish the National Practitioner Data Bank (NPDB) with all information reported to the national health care fraud and abuse data collection program on certain final adverse actions taken against health care providers, suppliers, and practitioners.

Requires the Secretary to establish a process to terminate the Healthcare Integrity and Protection Databank (HIPDB) and ensure that the information formerly collected in it is transferred to the NPDB.

(Sec. 6404) Reduces from three years to one year after the date of service the maximum period for submission of Medicare claims.

(Sec. 6405, as modified by Sec. 10604) Requires DME or home health services to be ordered by an enrolled Medicare eligible professional or physician. Authorizes the Secretary to extend these requirements to other Medicare items and services to reduce fraud, waste, and abuse.

(Sec. 6406) Authorizes the Secretary to disenroll, for up to one year, a Medicare enrolled physician or supplier that fails to maintain and provide access to written orders or requests for payment for DME, certification for home health services, or referrals for other items and services.

Authorizes the Secretary to exclude from participation in any federal health care program any individual or entity ordering, referring for furnishing, or certifying the need for an item or service that fails to provide adequate documentation to verify payment.

(Sec. 6407, as modified by Sec. 10605) Requires a physician, nurse practitioner, clinical nurse specialist, certified nurse-midwife, or physician assistant to have a face-to-face encounter with an individual before issuing a certification for home health services or DME.

Authorizes the Secretary to apply the same face-to-face encounter requirement to other items and services based upon a finding that doing so would reduce the risk of fraud, waste, and abuse. Applies the same requirement, as well, to physicians making certifications for home health services under Medicaid.

(Sec. 6408) Revises civil monetary penalties for making false statements or delaying inspections.

Applies specified enhanced sanctions and civil monetary penalties to MA or Part D plans that: (1) enroll individuals in an MA or Part D plan without their consent; (2) transfer an individual from one plan to another for the purpose of earning a commission; (3) fail to comply with marketing requirements and CMMS guidance; or (4) employ or contract with an individual or entity that commits a violation.

(Sec. 6409) Requires the Secretary to establish a self-referral disclosure protocol to enable health care providers and suppliers to disclose actual or potential violations of the physician self-referral law.

Authorizes the Secretary to reduce the amount due and owing for all violations of such law.

(Sec. 6410) Requires the Secretary to: (1) expand the number of areas to be included in round two of the competitive bidding program from 79 to 100 of the largest metropolitan statistical areas; and (2) use competitively bid prices in all areas by 2016.

(Sec. 6411) Requires states to establish contracts with one or more Recovery Audit Contractors (RACs), which shall identify underpayments and overpayments and recoup overpayments made for services provided under state Medicaid plans as well as state plan waivers.

Requires the Secretary to expand the RAC program to Medicare Parts C (Medicare+Choice) and D (Prescription Drug Program).

Subtitle F: Additional Medicaid Program Integrity Provisions

(Sec. 6501) Amends SSA title XIX (Medicaid) to require states to terminate individuals or entities (providers) from their Medicaid programs if they were terminated from Medicare or another state's Medicaid program.

(Sec. 6502) Requires Medicaid agencies to exclude individuals or entities from participating in Medicaid for a specified period of time if the entity or individual owns, controls, or manages an entity that: (1) has failed to repay overpayments during a specified period; (2) is suspended, excluded, or terminated from participation in any Medicaid program; or (3) is affiliated with an individual or entity that has been suspended, excluded, or terminated from Medicaid participation.

(Sec. 6503) Requires state Medicaid plans to require any billing agents, clearinghouses, or other alternate payees that submit claims on behalf of health care providers to register with the state and the Secretary.

(Sec. 6504) Requires states to submit data elements from the state mechanized claims processing and information retrieval system (under the Medicaid Statistical Information System) that the Secretary determines necessary for program integrity, program oversight, and administration.

Requires a Medicaid managed care entity contract to provide for maintenance of sufficient patient encounter data to identify the physician who delivers services to patients (as under current law) at a frequency and level of detail to be specified by the Secretary.

(Sec. 6505) Requires a state Medicaid plan to prohibit the state from making any payments for items or services under a Medicaid state plan or a waiver to any financial institution or entity located outside of the United States.

(Sec. 6506) Extends the period for states to recover overpayments from 60 days to one year after discovery of the overpayment. Declares that, when overpayments due to fraud are pending, state repayments of the federal portion of such overpayments shall not be due until 30 days after the date of the final administrative or judicial judgment on the matter.

(Sec. 6507) Requires state mechanized Medicaid claims processing and information retrieval systems to incorporate methodologies compatible with Medicare's National Correct Coding Initiative.

Subtitle G: Additional Program Integrity Provisions

(Sec. 6601) Amends the Employee Retirement Income Security Act of 1974 (ERISA) to prohibit employees and agents of multiple employer welfare arrangements (MEWAs), subject to criminal penalties, from making false statements in marketing materials regarding an employee welfare benefit plan's financial solvency, benefits, or regulatory status.

(Sec. 6603) Amends the Public Health Service Act to direct the Secretary to request NAIC to develop a model uniform report form for a private health insurance issuer seeking to refer suspected fraud and abuse to state insurance departments or other responsible state agencies for investigation.

(Sec. 6604) Amends ERISA to direct the Secretary of Labor to adopt regulatory standards and/or issue orders to subject MEWAs to state law relating to fraud and abuse.

(Sec. 6605) Authorizes the Secretary of Labor to: (1) issue cease-and-desist orders to shut down temporarily the operations of MEWAs conducting fraudulent activities or posing a serious threat to the public, until hearings can be completed; and (2) seize a plan's assets if it appears that the plan is in a financially hazardous condition.

(Sec. 6606) Directs the Secretary of Labor to require MEWAs which are not group health plans to register with the Department of Labor before operating in a state.

(Sec. 6607) Authorizes the Secretary of Labor to promulgate a regulation providing an evidentiary privilege that allows confidential communication among specified federal and state officials relating to investigation of fraud and abuse.

Subtitle H: Elder Justice Act

(Sec. 6702) Elder Justice Act of 2009. Amends SSA title XX (Block Grants to States for Social Services) with respect to elder abuse, neglect, and exploitation and their prevention. Requires the HHS Secretary to award grants and carry out activities that provide: (1) greater protection to those individuals seeking care in facilities that provide long-term care services and supports; and (2) greater incentives for individuals to train and seek employment at such facilities. Requires facility owners, operators, and certain employees to report suspected crimes committed at a facility.

Requires facility owners or operators also to: (1) submit to the Secretary and to the state written notification of an impending closure of a facility within 60 days before the closure; and (2) include a plan for transfer and adequate relocation of all residents.

Establishes an Elder Justice Coordinating Council.

Subtitle I: Sense of the Senate Regarding Medical Malpractice

(Sec. 6801) Expresses the sense of the Senate that: (1) health reform presents an opportunity to address issues related to medical malpractice and medical liability insurance; (2) states should be encouraged to develop and test alternative models to the existing civil litigation system; and (3) Congress should consider state demonstration projects to evaluate such alternatives.

Title VII: Improving Access to Innovative Medical Therapies

Subtitle A: Biologics Price Competition and Innovation

(Sec. 7002) Biologics Price Competition and Innovation Act of 2009. Amends the Public Health Service Act to allow a person to submit an application for licensure of a biological product based on its similarity to a licensed biological product (the reference product). Requires the Secretary to license the biological product if it is biosimilar to or interchangeable with the reference product.

Prohibits the Secretary from determining that a second or subsequent biological product is interchangeable with a reference product for any condition of use for specified periods based on the marketing of, and the presence or status of litigation involving, the first biosimilar biological product deemed interchangeable with the same reference product.

Prohibits the Secretary from making approval of an application under this Act effective until 12 years after the date on which the reference product was first licensed.

Subtitle B: More Affordable Medicine
for Children and Underserved Communities

(Sec. 7101) Expands the 340B drug discount program (a program limiting the cost of covered outpatient drugs to certain federal grantees) to allow participation as a covered entity by certain: (1) children's hospitals; (2) freestanding cancer hospitals; (3) critical access hospitals; (4) rural referral centers; and (5) sole community hospitals. Expands the program to include drugs used in connection with an inpatient or outpatient service by enrolled hospitals (currently, only outpatient drugs are covered under the program).

Prohibits enrolled hospitals from obtaining covered outpatient drugs through a group purchasing arrangement. Requires the Secretary to establish reasonable exceptions to such prohibition, including for drugs unavailable through the program and to facilitate generic substitution when a generic covered drug is available at a lower price.

Requires a hospital enrolled in the 340B drug discount program to issue a credit to a state Medicaid program for inpatient covered drugs provided to Medicaid recipients.

(Sec. 7102) Requires the Secretary to: (1) provide for improvements in compliance by manufacturers and covered entities with the requirements of the 340B drug discount program; and (2) establish and implement an administrative process for resolving claims by covered entities and manufacturers of violations of such requirements.

Requires manufacturers to offer each covered entity an opportunity to purchase covered drugs for purchase at or below the applicable ceiling price if such a drug is made available to any other purchaser at any price.

(Sec. 7103) Requires the Comptroller General to report to Congress on whether those individuals served by the covered entities under the 340B drug discount program are receiving optimal health care services.

Title VIII: CLASS Act

(Sec. 8002, as modified by Sec. 10801) Community Living Assistance Services and Supports Act or the CLASS Act. Establishes a national, voluntary insurance program for purchasing community living assistance services and supports (CLASS program) under which: (1) all employees are automatically enrolled, but are allowed to waive enrollment; (2) payroll deductions pay monthly premiums; and (3) benefits under a CLASS Independence Benefit Plan provide individuals with functional limitations with tools that will allow them to maintain their personal and financial independence and live in the community.

Title IX: Revenue Provisions

Subtitle A: Revenue Offset Provisions

(Sec. 9001, as modified by section 10901) Amends the Internal Revenue Code to impose an excise tax of 40% of the excess benefit from certain high cost employer-sponsored health coverage. Deems any amount which exceeds payment of $8,500 for an employee self-only coverage plan and $23,000 for employees with other than self-only coverage (family plans) as an excess benefit. Increases such amounts for certain retirees and employees who are engaged in high-risk professions (e.g., law enforcement officers, emergency medical first responders, or longshoremen). Imposes a penalty on employers and coverage providers for failure to calculate the proper amount of an excess benefit.

(Sec. 9002) Requires employers to include in the W-2 form of each employee the aggregate cost of applicable employer-sponsored group health coverage that is excludable from the employee's gross income (excluding the value of contributions to flexible spending arrangements).

(Sec. 9003) Restricts payments from health savings accounts, medical savings accounts, and health flexible spending arrangements for medications to prescription drugs or insulin.

(Sec. 9004) Increases to 20% the penalty for distributions from a health savings account or Archer medical savings account not used for qualified medical expenses.

(Sec. 9005, as modified by section 10902) Limits annual salary reduction contributions by an employee to a health flexible spending arrangement under a cafeteria plan to $2,500. Allows an annual inflation adjustment to such amount after 2011.

(Sec. 9006) Expands reporting requirements for payments of $600 or more to corporations (other than tax-exempt corporations).

(Sec. 9007, as modified by section 10903) Requires tax-exempt charitable hospitals to: (1) conduct a community health needs assessment every two years; (2) adopt a written financial assistance policy for patients who require financial assistance for hospital care; and (3) refrain from taking extraordinary collection actions against a patient until the hospital has made reasonable efforts to determine whether the patient is eligible for financial assistance. Imposes a penalty tax on hospitals who fail to comply with the requirements of this Act.

Requires the Secretary of the Treasury to report to Congress on information with respect to private tax-exempt, taxable, and government-owned hospitals regarding levels of charity care provided, bad debt expenses, unreimbursed costs, and costs for community benefit activities.

(Sec. 9008) Imposes an annual fee on the branded prescription drug sales exceeding $5 million of manufacturers and importers of such drugs beginning in 2010. Requires the HHS, VA, and DOD Secretaries to report to the Secretary of the Treasury on the total branded prescription drug sales within government programs within their departments.

(Sec. 9009, as modified by section 10904) Imposes an annual fee on the gross sales receipts exceeding $5 million of manufacturers and importers of certain medical devices beginning in 2011.

(Sec. 9010, as modified by section 10905) Imposes on any entity that provides health insurance for any United States health risk an annual fee beginning in 2011. Exempts entities whose net premiums written are not more than $25 million. Requires all entities subject to such fee to report to the Secretary of the Treasury on their net written premiums and imposes a penalty for failure to report.

(Sec. 9011) Requires the VA Secretary to study and report to Congress by December 31, 2012, on the effect of fees assessed by this Act on the cost of medical care provided to veterans and on veterans' access to medical devices and branded prescription drugs.

(Sec. 9012) Eliminates the tax deduction for expenses for determining the subsidy for employers who maintain prescription drug plans for Medicare Part D eligible retirees.

(Sec. 9013) Increases the adjusted gross income threshold for claiming the itemized deduction for medical expenses from 7.5% to 10% beginning after 2012. Retains the 7.5% threshold through 2016 for individual taxpayers who have attained age 65 before the close of an applicable taxable year.

(Sec. 9014) Imposes a limitation after December 31, 2012, of $500,000 on the deductibility of remuneration paid to officers, directors, employees, and service providers of health insurance issuers who derive at least 25% of their gross premiums from providing health insurance coverage that meets the minimum essential coverage requirements established by this Act.

(Sec. 9015, as modified by section 10906) Increases after December 31, 2012, the hospital insurance tax rate by .9% for individual taxpayers earning over $200,000 ($250,000 for married couples filing joint tax returns).

(Sec. 9016) Requires Blue Cross or Blue Shield organizations or other nonprofit organizations that provide health insurance to reimburse at least 85% of the cost of clinical services provided to their enrollees to be eligible for special tax benefits currently provided to such organizations.

Subtitle B: Other Provisions

(Sec. 9021) Excludes from gross income the value of certain health benefits provided to members of Indian tribes, including: (1) health services or benefits provided or purchased by IHS; (2) medical care provided by an Indian tribe or tribal organization to a member of an Indian tribe; (3) accident or health plan coverage provided by an Indian tribe or tribal organization for medical care to a member of an Indian tribe and dependents; and (4) any other medical care provided by an Indian tribe that supplements, replaces, or substitutes for federal programs.

(Sec. 9022) Establishes a new employee benefit cafeteria plan to be known as a Simple Cafeteria Plan, defined as a plan that: (1) is established and maintained by an employer with an average of 100 or fewer employees during a two-year period; (2) requires employers to make contributions or match employee contributions to the plan; (3) requires participating employees to have at least 1,000 hours of service for the preceding plan year; and (4) allows such employees to elect any benefit available under the plan.

(Sec. 9023) Allows a 50% tax credit for investment in any qualifying therapeutic discovery project, defined as a project that is designed to: (1) treat or prevent diseases by conducting pre-clinical activities, clinical trials, and clinical studies, or carrying out research projects to approve new drugs or other biologic products; (2) diagnose diseases or conditions to determine molecular factors related to diseases or conditions; or (3) develop a product, process, or technology to further the delivery or administration of therapeutics. Directs the Secretary of the Treasury to award grants for 50% of the investment in 2009 or 2010 in such a project, in lieu of the tax credit.

Title X: Strengthening Quality, Affordable Health Care for All Americans

Subtitle A: Provisions Relating to Title I

(Sec. 10101) Revises provisions of or related to Subtitles A, B, and C of Title I of this Act (as reflected in the summary of those provisions).

(Sec. 10104) Revises provisions of or related to Subtitle D of Title I of this Act (as reflected in the summary of those provisions). Makes changes to the False Claims Act related to the public disclosure bar on filing civil claims.

(Sec. 10105) Revises provisions of or related to Subtitles E, F, and G of Title I of this Act (as reflected in the summary of those provisions).

(Sec. 10108) Requires an offering employer to provide free choice vouchers to each qualified employee. Defines "offering employer" to mean any employer who offers minimum essential coverage to its employees consisting of coverage through an eligible employer-sponsored plan and who pays any portion of the costs of such plan. Defines "qualified employee" as an employee whose required contribution for such coverage and household income fall within a specified range. Requires: (1) a Health Insurance Exchange to credit the amount of any free choice voucher to the monthly premium of any qualified health plan in which the employee is enrolled; and (2) the offering employer to pay any amounts so credited to the Exchange. Excludes the amount of any free choice voucher from the gross income of the employee. Permits a deduction by employers for such costs.

(Sec. 10109) Amends the SSA to require the HHS Secretary to seek input to determine if there could be greater uniformity in financial and administrative health care activities and items.

Requires the Secretary to: (1) task the ICD-9-CM Coordination and Maintenance Committee to convene a meeting to receive input regarding and recommend revisions to the crosswalk between the Ninth and Tenth Revisions of the International Classification of Diseases; and (2) make appropriate revisions to such crosswalk.

Subtitle B: Provisions Relating to Title II

Part I: Medicaid and CHIP

(Sec. 10201) Revises provisions of Subtitles A through L of Title II of this Act (as reflected in the summary of those provisions).

Amends SSA title XIX (Medicaid) to set the FMAP for the state of Nebraska, with respect to all or any portion of a fiscal year that begins on or after January 1, 2017, at 100% (thus requiring the federal government to pay 100% of the cost of covering newly-eligible individuals in Nebraska).

Directs the Comptroller General to study and report to Congress on whether the development, recognition, or implementation of any specified health care quality guideline or other standards would result in the establishment of a new cause of action or claim.

(Sec. 10202) Creates a State Balancing Incentive Payments Program to increase the FMAP for states which offer home and community-based services as a long-term care alternative to nursing homes.

(Sec. 10203) Amends SSA title XXI (CHIP) to make appropriations for CHIP through FY2015 and revise other CHIP-related requirements.

Part II: Support for Pregnant and Parenting Teens and Women

(Sec. 10212) Requires the Secretary to establish a Pregnancy Assistance Fund for grants to states to assist pregnant and parenting teens and women.

(Sec. 10214) Authorizes appropriations for FY2010-FY2019.

Part III: Indian Health Care Improvement

(Sec. 10221) Enacts into law the Indian Health Care Improvement Reauthorization and Extension Act of 2009 (S. 1790), as reported by the Committee on Indian Affairs of the Senate in December 2009.

Amends the Indian Health Care Improvement Act, as amended by the Indian Health Care Improvement Reauthorization and Extension Act of 2009, to make an exception to the requirement that a national Community Health Aide

Program exclude dental health aide therapist services. Declares that the exclusion of dental health aide therapist services from services covered under the national program shall not apply where an Indian tribe or tribal organization, located in a state (other than Alaska) in which state law authorizes the use of dental health aide therapist services or midlevel dental health provider services, elects to supply such services in accordance with state law.

Subtitle C: Provisions Relating to Title III

(Sec. 10301) Revises provisions of Subtitles A through G of Title III of this Act (as reflected in the summary of those provisions).

(Sec. 10323) Amends SSA title XVIII (Medicare) to deem eligible for Medicare coverage certain individuals exposed to environmental health hazards.

Directs the Secretary to establish a pilot program for care of certain individuals residing in emergency declaration areas.

Amends SSA title XX (Block Grants to States for Social Services) to direct the Secretary to establish a program for early detection of certain medical conditions related to environmental health hazards. Makes appropriations for FY2012-FY2019.

(Sec. 10324) Establishes floors: (1) on the area wage index for hospitals in frontier states; (2) on the area wage adjustment factor for hospital outpatient department services in frontier states; and (3) for practice expense index for services furnished in frontier states.

(Sec. 10325) Revises the SNF prospective payment system to delay specified changes until FY2011.

(Sec. 10326) Directs the Secretary to conduct separate pilot programs, for specified kinds of hospitals and hospice programs, to test the implementation of a value-based purchasing program for payments to the provider.

(Sec. 10327) Authorizes an additional incentive payment under the physician quality reporting system in 2011 through 2014 to eligible professionals who report quality measures to CMMS via a qualified Maintenance of Certification program. Eliminates the Medicare Advantage Regional Plan Stabilization Fund.

(Sec. 10328) Requires Medicare Part D prescription drug plans to include a comprehensive review of medications as part of their medication therapy management programs. Requires automatic quarterly enrollment of qualified beneficiaries, with an allowance for them to opt out.

(Sec. 10329) Requires the Secretary to develop a methodology to measure health plan value.

(Sec. 10330) Directs the Secretary to develop a plan to modernize CMMS computer and data systems.

(Sec. 10331) Requires the Secretary to: (1) develop a Physician Compare Internet website with information on physicians enrolled in the Medicare program and other eligible professionals who participate in the Physician Quality Reporting Initiative; and (2) implement a plan to make information on physician performance public through Physician Compare, particularly quality and patient experience measures.

Authorizes the Secretary to provide financial incentives to Medicare beneficiaries furnished services by high quality physicians.

(Sec. 10332) Directs the Secretary to make available to qualified entities standardized extracts of Medicare claims data for the evaluation of the performance of service providers and suppliers.

(Sec. 10333) Amends the Public Health Service Act to authorize the Secretary to award grants to eligible entities to support community-based collaborative care networks for low-income populations.

(Sec. 10334) Transfers the Office of Minority Health to the Office of the Secretary. Authorizes appropriations for FY2011-FY2016.

Establishes individual offices of minority health within HHS.

Redesignates the National Center on Minority Health and Health Disparities in the National Institutes of Health as the National Institute on Minority Health and Health Disparities.

(Sec. 10336) Directs the Comptroller General to study and report to Congress on the impact on Medicare beneficiary access to high-quality dialysis services of including specified oral drugs furnished to them for the treatment of end state renal disease in the related bundled prospective payment system.

Subtitle D: Provisions Relating to Title IV

(Sec. 10401) Revises provisions of or related to Subtitles A, B, C, D, and E of Title IV of this Act (as reflected in the summary of those provisions).

(Sec. 10407) Catalyst to Better Diabetes Care Act of 2009—Requires the Secretary to prepare biennially a national diabetes report card and, to the extent possible, one for each state.

Requires the Secretary, acting through the Director of CDC, to: (1) promote the education and training of physicians on the importance of birth and death certificate data and on how to properly complete these documents; (2) encourage state adoption of the latest standard revisions of birth and death certificates; and (3) work with states to reengineer their vital statistics systems in order to provide cost-effective, timely, and accurate vital systems data. Allows the Secretary to promote improvements to the collection of diabetes mortality data.

Directs the Secretary to conduct a study of the impact of diabetes on the practice of medicine in the United States and the level of diabetes medical education that should be required prior to licensure, board certification, and board recertification.

(Sec. 10408) Requires the Secretary to award grants to eligible employers to provide their employees with access to comprehensive workplace wellness programs.

(Sec. 10409) Cures Acceleration Network Act of 2009—Amends the Public Health Service Act to require the Secretary, acting through the Director of the

National Institutes of Health (NIH), to implement the Cures Acceleration Network under which grants and contracts will be awarded to accelerate the development of high need cures. Defines "high need cure" as a drug, biological product, or device: (1) that is a priority to diagnose, mitigate, prevent, or treat harm from any disease or condition; and (2) for which the incentives of the commercial market are unlikely to result in its adequate or timely development. Establishes a Cures Acceleration Network Review Board.

(Sec. 10410) Establishing a Network of Health-Advancing National Centers of Excellence for Depression Act of 2009 or the ENHANCED Act of 2009— Requires the Secretary, acting through the Administrator of the Substance Abuse and Mental Health Services Administration, to: (1) award grants to establish national centers of excellence for depression; and (2) designate one such center as a coordinating center. Requires the coordinating center to establish and maintain a national, publicly available database to improve prevention programs, evidence-based interventions, and disease management programs for depressive disorders using data collected from the national centers.

(Sec. 10411) Congenital Heart Futures Act—Authorizes the Secretary, acting through the Director of CDC, to: (1) enhance and expand infrastructure to track the epidemiology of congenital heart disease and to organize such information into the National Congenital Heart Disease Surveillance System; or (2) award a grant to an eligible entity to undertake such activities.

Authorizes the Director of the National Heart, Lung, and Blood Institute to expand, intensify, and coordinate research and related Institute activities on congenital heart disease.

(Sec. 10412) Reauthorizes appropriations for grants for public access defibrillation programs. Requires an information clearinghouse to increase public access to defibrillation in schools established under such program to be administered by an organization that has substantial expertise in pediatric education, pediatric medicine, and electrophysiology and sudden death.

(Sec. 10413) Young Women's Breast Health Education and Awareness Requires Learning Young Act of 2009 or the EARLY Act—Requires the Secretary, acting through the Director of CDC, to conduct: (1) a national education campaign to increase awareness of young women's knowledge regarding breast health and breast cancer; (2) an education campaign among physicians and other health care professionals to increase awareness of breast health of young women; and (3) prevention research on breast cancer in younger women.

Requires the Secretary, acting through the Director of NIH, to conduct research to develop and validate new screening tests and methods for prevention and early detection of breast cancer in young women.

Directs the Secretary to award grants for the provision of health information to young women diagnosed with breast cancer and pre-neoplastic breast diseases.

Subtitle E: Provisions Relating to Title V

(Sec. 10501) Revises provisions of or related to Title V of this Act (as reflected in the summary of those provisions).

Requires the Secretary, acting through the Director of CDC, to establish a national diabetes prevention program targeted at adults at high risk for diabetes.

Directs the Secretary to develop a Medicare prospective payment system for payment for services furnished by federally qualified health centers.

Requires the Secretary, acting through the Administrator of the HRSA, to establish a grant program to assist accredited schools of allopathic or osteopathic medicine in: (1) recruiting students most likely to practice medicine in underserved rural communities; (2) providing rural-focused training and experience; and (3) increasing the number of recent allopathic and osteopathic medical school graduates who practice in underserved rural communities.

Directs the Secretary, acting through the Administrator of HRSA, to award grants or enter into contracts with eligible entities to provide training to graduate medical residents in preventive medicine specialties.

Reauthorizes appropriations for public health workforce activities.

Revises provisions related to fulfillment of service obligations under the National Health Service Corps related to half-time clinical practice and teaching.

(Sec. 10502) Authorizes appropriations to HHS for debt service on, or direct construction or renovation of, a health care facility that provides research, inpatient tertiary care, or outpatient clinical services and that meets certain requirements, including that it is critical for the provision of greater access to health care within the state.

(Sec. 10503) Establishes a Community Health Center Fund to provide for expanded and sustained national investment in community health centers. Authorizes appropriations to such Fund.

(Sec. 10504) Requires the Secretary, acting through the Administrator of HRSA, to establish a demonstration project to provide access to comprehensive health care services to the uninsured at reduced fees.

Subtitle F: Provisions Relating to Title VI

(Sec. 10601) Revises provisions of Subtitles A through E of Title IV of this Act (as reflected in the summary of those provisions).

(Sec. 10606) Directs the U.S. Sentencing Commission to amend the Federal Sentencing Guidelines to provide two-level, three-level, and four-level increases in the offense level for any defendant convicted of a federal health care offense relating to a Government health care program of a loss between $1 million and $7 million, between $7 million and $20 million, and at least $20 million, respectively.

Provides that a person need not have actual knowledge of the prohibition against health care fraud nor specific intent to violate it in order to commit health care fraud.

Expands the scope of violations constituting a federal health care offense.

Amends the Civil Rights of Institutionalized Persons Act to authorize the Attorney General to require access to an institution by subpoena to investigate conditions depriving residents of specified constitutional or federal rights.

(Sec. 10607) Authorizes the Secretary to award demonstration grants to states for the development, implementation, and evaluation of alternatives to current tort litigation for resolving disputes over injuries allegedly caused by health care providers or health care organizations.

(Sec. 10608) Amends the Public Health Service Act to extend medical malpractice coverage to free clinics by deeming their officers, employees, board members, and contractors to be employees of the Public Health Service.

(Sec. 10609) Amends the Federal, Drug, and Cosmetic Act to provide that, if the proposed labeling of a drug that is the subject of an application for approval as a new drug differs from the listed drug due to labeling revision, the drug that is the subject of such application shall be eligible for approval and shall not be considered misbranded if certain requirements are met.

Subtitle G: Provisions Relating to Title VIII

(Sec. 10801) Revises provisions of or related to Title VIII of this Act (as reflected in the summary of those provisions).

Subtitle H: Provisions Relating to Title IX

(Sec. 10901) Revises provisions of or related to Title IX of this Act (as reflected in the summary of those provisions).

(Sec. 10907) Amends the Internal Revenue Code to impose a 10% excise tax on any amount paid for indoor tanning services on or after July 1, 2010. Exempts phototherapy services performed by a licensed medical professional from the definition of "indoor tanning services."

(Sec. 10908) Excludes from gross income any payments under the National Health Service Corps Loan Repayment Program and any other state loan repayment or forgiveness programs intended to increase the availability of health care services in underserved or health professional shortage areas.

(Sec. 10909) Increases from $10,000 to $13,170 the dollar limitation on: (1) the tax credit for adoption expenses; and (2) the tax exclusion for employer-provided adoption assistance. Allows an inflation adjustment to such limitation after 2010. Makes such credit refundable. Extends through 2011 the general terminating date of the Economic Growth and Tax Relief Reconciliation Act of 2001 with respect to such credit and exclusion.

After both chambers of Congress approved the original measure, lawmakers turned to a package that included numerous revisions demanded by the House. That legislation was written under special budget "reconciliation" rules that protected the changes from a Senate filibuster.

Most of the provisions in the second bill were aimed at reducing the legislation's financial burden for individuals and local governments. The package also eliminated a handful of special deals that had been included to secure the original bill's passage in the Senate but that had stirred a public outcry, such as the "Cornhusker Kickback."

Highlights of the reconciliation bill include increased funding for states to provide Medicaid services and more generous subsidies for middle-class families to buy coverage. The measure also reduced the excise tax on high-value insurance policies and made up for the lost revenue by imposing a new Medicare tax on the wealthy.

Following is a House committee report that lays out its provisions.

Prepared by Committees on Ways & Means,
Energy & Commerce, and Education & Labor,
March 23, 2010

* * *

H.R. 4872
Title:
The Health Care & Education Reconciliation Act

The Health Care & Education Reconciliation Act

Title I: Coverage, Medicare, Medicaid and Revenues

Subtitle A: Coverage

Sec. 1001. Tax Credits. Improves the financing for premiums and cost sharing for individuals with incomes up to 400% of the federal poverty level. Subsection (a) improves tax credits to make premiums more affordable as a percent of income; and subsection (b) improves support for cost sharing, focusing on those with incomes below 250% of the federal poverty level. Starting in 2019, constrains the growth in tax credits if premiums are growing faster than the consumer price index, unless spending is more than 10% below current Congressional Budget Office (CBO) projections.

Sec. 1002. Individual responsibility. Modifies the assessment that individuals who choose to remain uninsured pay in three ways: (a) exempts the income below the filing threshold, (b) lowers the flat payment from $495 to $325 in 2015 and from $750 to $695 in 2016 and (c) raises the percent of income that is an alternative payment amount from 0.5 to 1.0% in 2014, 1.0 to 2.0% in 2015, and 2.0 to 2.5% for 2016 and subsequent years to make the assessment more progressive.

Sec. 1003. Employer responsibility. Improves the transition to the employer responsibility policy for employers with 50 or more full-time equivalent workers (FTE) by subtracting the first 30 full-time employees from the payment calculation (e.g., a firm with 51 workers that does not offer coverage will pay an amount equal to 51 minus 30, or 21 times the applicable per employee payment amount). The provision also changes the applicable payment amount for firms with more than 50 FTEs that do not offer coverage to $2,000 per full-time employee. It also eliminates the assessment for workers in a waiting period, while maintaining the 90-day limit on the length of any waiting period beginning in 2014.

Sec. 1004. Income definitions. Modifies the definition of income that is used for purposes of subsidy eligibility and the individual responsibility requirement.

The modifications conform the income definition to information that is currently reported on the Form 1040 and to the present law income tax return filing thresholds. The provision also extends the exclusion from gross income for employer provided health coverage for adult children up to age 26.

Sec. 1005. Implementation funding. Provides $1 billion to the Secretary of Health and Human Services to finance the administrative costs of implementing health insurance reform.

Subtitle B: Medicare

Sec. 1101. Closing the Medicare prescription drug "doughnut hole." Provides a $250 rebate for all Medicare Part D enrollees who enter the doughnut hole in 2010. Builds on pharmaceutical manufacturers' 50% discount on brand-name drugs beginning in 2011 to completely close the doughnut hole with 75% discounts on brand-name and generic drugs by 2020. Reduces the growth rate of the Part D spending threshold for catastrophic benefits between 2014 and 2019, providing additional benefits for seniors with high drug costs.

Sec. 1102. Medicare Advantage payments. Freezes Medicare Advantage payments in 2011. Beginning in 2012, the provision reduces Medicare Advantage benchmarks relative to current levels. Benchmarks will vary from 95% of Medicare spending in high-spending areas to 115% of Medicare spending in low-cost areas. The changes will be phased-in over 3, 5 or 7 years, depending on the level of payment reductions. The provision creates an incentive system to increase payments to high-quality plans by at least 5%. It also extends CMS authority to adjust risk scores in Medicare Advantage for observed differences in coding patterns relative to fee-for-service.

Sec. 1103. Savings from limits on MA plan administrative costs. Ensures Medicare Advantage plans spend at least 85% of revenue on medical costs or activities that improve quality of care, rather than profit and overhead.

Sec. 1104 Disproportionate share hospital (DSH) payments. Advances Medicare disproportionate share hospital cuts to begin in fiscal year 2014 but lowers the ten-year reduction by $3 billion.

Sec. 1105. Market basket updates. Revises the hospital market basket reduction that is in addition to the productivity adjustment as follows: -0.3 in FY14 and -0.75 in FY17, FY18 and FY19. Removes Senate provision that eliminates the additional market basket for hospitals based on coverage levels. Providers affected are inpatient hospitals, long-term care hospitals, inpatient rehabilitation facilities, psychiatric hospitals and outpatient hospitals.

Sec. 1106. Physician ownership-referral. Changes to December 31, 2010 the date after which physician ownership of hospitals to which they self refer is prohibited and provides a limited exception to the growth restrictions for grandfathered physician owned hospitals that treat the highest percentage of Medicaid patients in their county (and are not the sole hospital in a county).

Sec. 1107. Payment for imaging services. Sets the assumed utilization rate at

75 percent for the practice expense portion of advance diagnostic imaging services.

Sec. 1108. PE GPCI adjustment for 2010.

Sec. 1109. Payment for qualifying hospitals. Provides $400 million for fiscal years 2011 and 2012 for additional payments to hospitals located in the bottom quartile of counties ranked by Medicare spending on benefits per enrollee.

Subtitle C: Medicaid

Sec. 1201. Federal funding for states. Strikes the provision for a permanent 100% federal matching rate for Nebraska for the Medicaid costs of newly eligible individuals. Provides federal Medicaid matching payments for the costs of services to expansion populations at the following rates: 100% in 2014, 2015, and 2016; 95% in 2017; 94% in 2018; 93% in 2019; and 90% thereafter. In the case of expansion states, reduces the state share of the costs of covering nonpregnant childless adults by 50% in 2014, 60% in 2015; 70% in 2016; 80% in 2017, 90% in 2018. In 2019 and thereafter, expansion states would bear the same state share of the costs of covering nonpregnant childless adults as non-expansion states (e.g., 7% in 2019, 10% thereafter).

Sec. 1202. Payments to primary care physicians. Requires that Medicaid payment rates to primary care physicians for furnishing primary care services be no less than 100% of Medicare payment rates in 2013 and 2014 (the first year of the Senate bill's Medicaid coverage expansion to all individuals with incomes under 133% of poverty). Provides 100% federal funding for the incremental costs to States of meeting this requirement.

Sec. 1203. Disproportionate share hospital payments. Lowers the reduction in federal Medicaid DSH payments from $18.1 billion to $14.1 billion and advances the reductions to begin in fiscal year 2014. Directs the Secretary to develop a methodology for reducing federal DSH allotments to all states in order to achieve the mandated reductions. Extends trhough FY 2013 the federal DSH allotment for a state that has a $0 allotment after FY 2011.

Sec. 1204. Funding for the territories. Increases federal funding in the Senate bill for Puerto Rico, Virgin Islands, Guam, American Samoa, and the Northern Marianas Islands by $2 billion. Raises the caps on federal Medicaid funding for each of the territories. Allows each territory to elect to operate a Health Benefits Exchange.

Sec. 1205. Delay in Community First Choice Option. Postpones from October 1, 2010 until October 1, 2011 the effective date of the option established for State Medicaid programs to cover attendant care services and supports for individuals who require an institutional level of care.

Sec. 1206. Drug rebates for new formulations of existing drugs. For purposes of applying the additional rebate, narrows the definition of a new formulation of a drug to a line extension of a single source or innovator multiple source drug that is an oral solid dosage form of the drug.

Subtitle D: Reducing Fraud, Waste, and Abuse

Sec. 1301. Community mental health centers. Establishes new requirements for community mental health centers that provide Medicare partial hospitalization services in order to prevent fraud and abuse.

Sec. 1302. Medicare prepayment medical review limitations. Streamlines procedures to conduct Medicare prepayment reviews to facilitate additional reviews designed to reduce fraud and abuse.

Sec. 1303. Funding to fight fraud, waste and abuse. Increases funding for the Health Care Fraud and Abuse Control Fund by $250 million over the next decade. Indexes funds to fight Medicaid fraud based on the increase in the Consumer Price Index.

Sec. 1304. 90-day period of enhanced oversight for initial claims of DME suppliers. Requires a 90-day period to withhold payment and conduct enhances oversight in cases where the HHS Secretary identifies a significant risk of fraud among DME suppliers.

Subtitle E: Revenues

Sec. 1401. High-cost plan excise tax. Reduces the revenue collected by the tax by 80 percent. This is achieved by: delaying the application of the tax until 2018, which gives the plans time to implement and realize the cost savings of reform; increasing the dollar thresholds to $10,200 for single coverage and $27,500 for family coverage ($11,850 and $30,950 for retirees and employees in high risk professions); excluding stand-alone dental and vision plans from the tax; and permitting an employer to reduce the cost of the coverage when applying the tax if the employer's age and gender demographics are not representative of the age and gender demographics of a national risk pool. Under the modified provision, the dollar thresholds are indexed to inflation and the dollar thresholds are automatically increased in 2018 if CBO is wrong in its forecast of the premium inflation rate between now and 2018.

Sec. 1402. Unearned income Medicare contribution. Modifies the Medicare contribution to include net investment income in the taxable base. Currently, the Medicare contribution does not apply to net investment income. The Medicare contribution on net investment income does not apply if modified adjusted gross income is less that $250,000 in the case of a joint return, or $200,000 in the case of a single return. Net investment income is interest, dividends, royalties, rents, gross income from a trade or business involving passive activities, and net gain from disposition of property (other than property held in a trade or business). Net investment income is reduced by properly allocable deductions to such income.

Sec. 1403. Delay of the annual limitation on contributions to a health flexible spending account. Delays the provision by two years until 2013.

Sec. 1404. Brand name pharmaceuticals. Delays the industry fee on sales of brand name pharmaceuticals for use in government health programs by one year to 2011, and increases revenue raised by the fee by $4.8 billion.

Sec. 1405. Excise tax on medical device manufacturers. Delays the tax by two years to 2013 and converts the industry fee to an excise tax on the sale of medical devices by manufacturers and importers at a rate of 2.3 percent. Exempts from the tax: eyeglasses, contact lenses, hearing aids, and any device specified by the Secretary of the Treasury that is of a type that is generally purchased by the public at retail for individual use.

Sec. 1406. Health insurance providers. Delays the fee by 3 years to 2014 and modifies the annual industry fee for revenue neutrality. In the case of tax-exempt insurance providers, provides that only 50 percent of their net premiums that relate to their tax-exempt status are taken into account in calculating the fee. Provides exemptions for voluntary employee benefit associations (VEBAs) and nonprofit providers more than 80 percent of whose revenues is received from Social Security Act programs that target low income, elderly, or disabled persons.

Sec. 1407. Delay of elimination of deduction for expenses allocable to Medicare Part D subsidy. Delays the provision by two years to 2013.

Sec. 1408. Elimination of unintended application of cellulosic biofuel producer credit. Adds an additional revenue provision. In 2008, Congress enacted a $1.01 per gallon tax credit for the production of biofuel from cellulosic feedstocks in order to encourage the development of new production capacity for biofuels that are not derived from food source materials. Congress is aware that some taxpayers are seeking to claim the cellulosic biofuel tax credit for unprocessed fuels, such as black liquor. The provision would limit eligibility for the tax credit to processed fuels (i.e., fuels that could be used in a car engine or in a home heating application).

Sec. 1409. Codification of economic substance doctrine and penalties. Adds an additional revenue provision. The economic substance doctrine is a judicial doctrine that has been used by the courts to deny tax benefits when the transaction generating these tax benefits lacks economic substance. The courts have not applied the economic substance doctrine uniformly. The provision would clarify the manner in which the economic substance doctrine should be applied by the courts and would impose a penalty on understatements attributable to a transaction lacking economic substance.

Sec. 1410. Time for payment of corporate estimated taxes. Provides for a one-time adjustment to corporate estimated taxes for payments made during calendar year 2014.

Subtitle F: Other Provisions

Sec. 1501. Trade Adjustment Assistance for communities. Appropriates $500 million a year for fiscal years 2010 through 2014 in the Community College and Career Training Grant program for community colleges to develop and improve educational or career training programs. Ensures that each state receives at least 0.5 percent of the total funds appropriated.

Title II: Health, Education, Labor and Pensions

Subtitle A: Education

Section 2001. Short title; references. Provides that this subtitle may be cited as the "SAFRA Act," and that, except as otherwise provided, whenever an amendment to, or repeal of, a section or other provision, the reference shall be considered to be made to a section or other provision of the Higher Education Act of 1965.

Part I: Investing in Students and Families

Section 2101. Federal Pell Grants. Amends the Higher Education Act to include mandatory funding for the Pell Grant. This provides additional mandatory funding to augment funds appropriated to increase the federal maximum Pell Grant award by the change in the Consumer Price Index. The mandatory component of the funding is determined by inflating the previous year's total and subtracting the maximum award provided for in the appropriations act for the previous year or $4860, whichever is greater. Beginning in 2018–2019 academic year, the maximum Pell award will be at the 2017–2018 level.

Section 2102. College Access Challenge Grant Program. This section amends section 786 of the Higher Education Act by authorizing and appropriating $150 million for fiscal years 2010 through 2014 for the College Access Challenge Grant program created under the College Cost Reduction and Access Act of 2007. Provides that the allotment for each State under this section for a fiscal year shall not be an amount that is less that 1.0 percent of the total amount appropriated for a fiscal year.

Section 2103. Investment in Historically Black Colleges and Universities and Minority Serving Institutions. This section amends section 371(b) of the Higher Education Act by extending funding for programs under this section created under the College Cost Reduction and Access Act of 2007 for programs at Historically Black Colleges and Universities and minority-serving institutions through 2019, including programs that help low-income students attain degrees in the fields of science, technology, engineering or mathematics by the following annual amounts: $100 million to Hispanic Serving Institutions, $85 million to Historically Black Colleges and Universities, $15 million to Predominantly Black

Institutions, $30 million to Tribal Colleges and Universities, $15 million to Alaska, Hawaiian Native Institutions, $5 million to Asian American and Pacific Islander Institutions, and $5 million to Native American non-tribal serving institutions.

Part II: Student Loan Reform

Section 2201. Termination of Federal Family Education Loan Appropriations. This section terminates the authority to make or insure any additional loans in the Federal Family Education Loan program after June 30, 2010.

Section 2202. Termination of Federal Loan Insurance Program. This section is a conforming amendment with regard to the termination of the FFEL program, limiting federal insurance to those loans in the Federal Family Education Loan program for loans first disbursed prior to July 1, 2010.

Section 2203. Termination of the applicable interest rates. This section makes a conforming amendment with regard to the termination of the FFEL program limiting interest rate applicability to Stafford, Consolidation, and PLUS loans to those loans made before July 1, 2010.

Section 2204. Termination of federal payments to reduce student interest costs. This section makes a conforming amendment with regard to the termination of the FFEL program by limiting subsidy payments to lenders for those loans for which the first disbursement is made before July 1, 2010.

Section 2205. Termination of the FFEL PLUS Loans. This section makes a conforming change with regard to the termination of the FFEL program for federal PLUS loans by prohibiting further FFEL origination of loans after July 1, 2010.

Section 2206. Federal Consolidation Loans. This section makes conforming changes with regard to the termination of the FFEL program for federal consolidation loans. This section also provides that, for a 1 year period, borrowers who have loans under both the Direct Lending program and the FFEL program, or who have loans under either program as well as loans that have been sold to the Secretary, may consolidate such loans under the Direct Lending program regardless of whether such borrowers have entered repayment on such loans.

Section 2207. Termination of the unsubsidized Stafford loans for middle-income borrowers. This section makes conforming changes with regards to the termination of the FFEL program for Unsubsidized Stafford loans by prohibiting further FFEL origination of loans after July 1, 2010.

Section 2208. Termination of special allowances. This section makes conforming changes with regards to the termination of the FFEL program by limiting special allowance payments to lenders under the FFEL program to loans first disbursed before July 1, 2010.

Section 2209. Origination of Direct Loans at institutions outside the United States. This section provides for the origination of federal Direct Loans at institutions located outside of the United States, through a financial institution designated by the Secretary.

Section 2210. Conforming amendments. This section makes conforming technical changes with regard to the termination of FFEL program for Department of Education agreements with Direct Lending institutions.

Section 2211. Terms and conditions of loans. This section makes conforming technical changes with regard to the termination of the FFEL program to clarify the terms and conditions of Direct Loans.

Section 2212. Contracts. This section directs the Secretary to award contracts for servicing federal Direct Loans to eligible non-profit servicers. In addition, this section provides that for the first 100,000 borrower loan accounts, the Secretary shall establish a separate pricing tier. Specifies that the Secretary is to allocate the loan accounts of 100,000 borrowers to each eligible non-profit servicer. The section also permits the Secretary to reallocate, increase, reduce or terminate an eligible non-profit servicer. In addition, this section appropriates mandatory funds to the Secretary to be obligated for administrative costs of servicing contracts with eligible non-profit servicers. This section also requires the Secretary to provide technical assistance to institutions of high education participating or seeking to participate in the Direct Lending program. This section appropriates $50 million for fiscal 2010 to pay for this technical assistance. Additionally, this section authorizes the Secretary to provide payments to loan servicers for retaining jobs at locations in the United States where such servicers were operating on January 1, 2010. This section appropriates $25,000,000 for each of fiscal years 2010 and 2011 for such purpose.

Section 2213. Income-Based Repayment. The section amends the Income-Based Repayment program to cap student loan payments of new borrowers after July 1, 2014 to 10% of adjusted income, from 15%, and to forgive remaining balances after 20 years of repayment, from 25 years.

Subtitle B: Health

Sec. 2301. Insurance Reforms. Extends the prohibition of lifetime limits, prohibition on rescissions, limitations on excessive waiting periods, and a requirement to provide coverage for non-dependent children up to age 26 to all existing health insurance plans starting six months after enactment. For group health plans, prohibits pre-existing condition exclusions in 2014, restricts annual limits beginning six months after enactment, and prohibits them starting in 2014. For coverage of non-dependent children prior to 2014, the requirement on group health plans is limited to those adult children without an employer offer of coverage.

Sec. 2302. Drugs purchased by covered entities. Repeals H.R. 3590's 340B expansion to inpatient drugs and exemptions to GPO exclusion. Exempts orphan drugs from required discounts for new 340B entities.

Sec. 2303. Community health centers. Increases mandatory funding for community health centers to $11 billion over five years (FY2011–FY 2015).

ACKNOWLEDGMENTS

This book is the work of *Washington Post* reporters who covered and analyzed the health-care legislation and its political fallout as the bills made their way through Congress: Dan Balz, David Brown, Ceci Connolly, Amy Goldstein, David S. Hilzenrath, Alec MacGillis, Lori Montgomery and Shailagh Murray, joined by Howard Gleckman of Kaiser Health News.

It was edited by David Finkel, Mary Hadar, Steve Luxenberg and Frances Stead Sellers, with strong support from Kevin Merida.

Carrie Camillo was the copy editor, with assistance from Kelly Johnson.

Alice Crites and Madonna Lebling provided research support.

Laura Stanton and Karen Yourish composed the graphics, edited by Larry Nista.

We owe much to the guidance of many health policy experts in think tanks, congressional offices, government agencies, universities, trade associations and consulting firms.

Finally, we are grateful for the thoughtful editorial input of John Fairhall of Kaiser Health News, an independent news service of the Henry J. Kaiser Family Foundation. Candy Lee provided her business acumen at *The Post* and at PublicAffairs Lindsay Jones and Melissa Raymond were the ideal publishing partners.

* * *

The account of the health-care debate by Ceci Connolly is based on interviews with more than five dozen White House officials, lawmakers, Catholic bishops, lobbyists, corporate executives, union leaders and their aides. Most of the interviews were conducted on the record, but a few sources were granted anonymity to discuss sensitive negotiations. All events described in the narrative were either witnessed or confirmed by at least two sources.

The guide that forms the book's second section, What It Means for Us All, is based on a close reading of the law's language, informed by the insights of the many health-care experts mentioned above. While the authors benefit from knowledge gained from a year of following the health-care debate, what you hold in your hands is freshly reported in the weeks immediately following the law's enactment.

INDEX

PublicAffairs is a publishing house founded in 1997. It is a tribute to the standards, values, and flair of three persons who have served as mentors to countless reporters, writers, editors, and book people of all kinds, including me.

I. F. STONE, proprietor of *I. F. Stone's Weekly*, combined a commitment to the First Amendment with entrepreneurial zeal and reporting skill and became one of the great independent journalists in American history. At the age of eighty, Izzy published *The Trial of Socrates*, which was a national bestseller. He wrote the book after he taught himself ancient Greek.

BENJAMIN C. BRADLEE was for nearly thirty years the charismatic editorial leader of *The Washington Post*. It was Ben who gave the *Post* the range and courage to pursue such historic issues as Watergate. He supported his reporters with a tenacity that made them fearless and it is no accident that so many became authors of influential, best-selling books.

ROBERT L. BERNSTEIN, the chief executive of Random House for more than a quarter century, guided one of the nation's premier publishing houses. Bob was personally responsible for many books of political dissent and argument that challenged tyranny around the globe. He is also the founder and longtime chair of Human Rights Watch, one of the most respected human rights organizations in the world.

. . .

For fifty years, the banner of Public Affairs Press was carried by its owner Morris B. Schnapper, who published Gandhi, Nasser, Toynbee, Truman, and about 1,500 other authors. In 1983, Schnapper was described by *The Washington Post* as "a redoubtable gadfly." His legacy will endure in the books to come.

Peter Osnos, *Founder and Editor-at-Large*